To Matt &
Alison,

SCAR TISSUE

Glad to have met
you,
Asaf

Malibu 5.2013

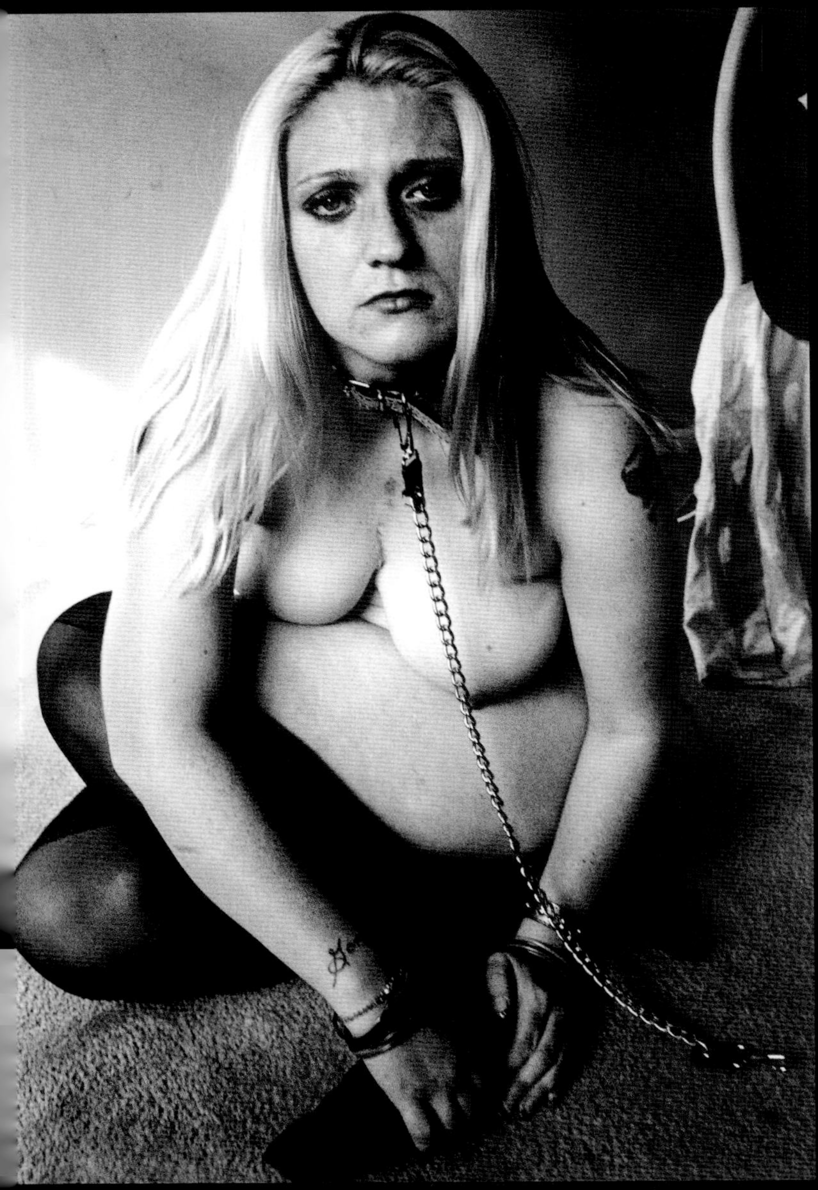

Sassy

Assaf Pocker

SCAR TISSUE

*

*

*

Nazraeli Press

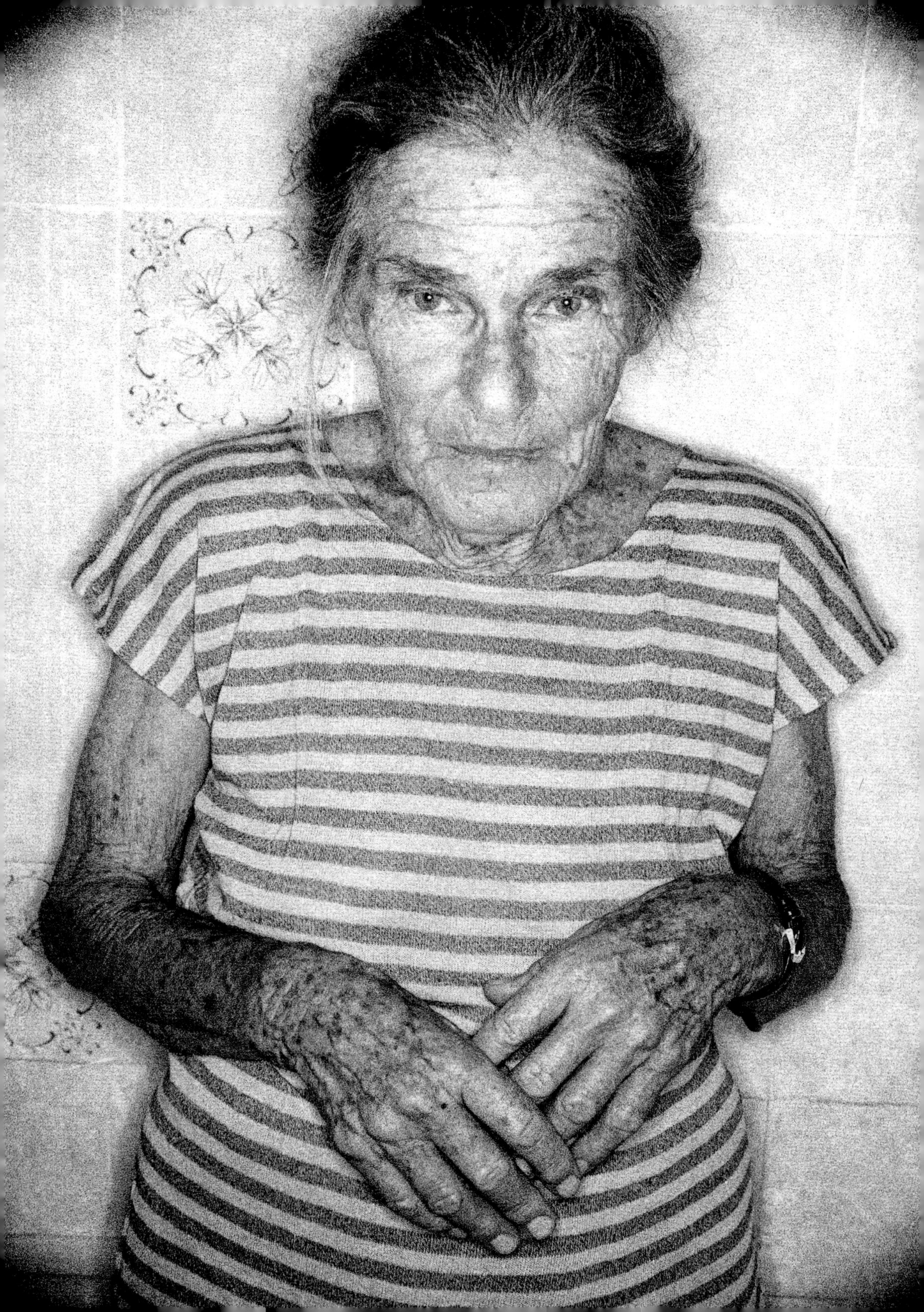

INTRODUCTION BY Renée T. Coulombe, PhD

"I can't tell you that I learned anything new in this process," he says, languidly chopping tomatoes in my kitchen. We've been here before, in this kitchen, in this conversation, tossing around the meaning of pain. We started talking about *Scar Tissue* from our very first conversations several years ago, mostly about the process, the journey. "What I learned wasn't knowledge that I didn't already have, but the degree, the level, the level of experience. It was very profound to see that."

Assaf and I have met for months now – talking, photographing, laughing and, more often than not crying together, telling stories about the lives whose intersections make up the pages that follow. This book is a story, but it is hundreds of stories. The kinds of stories that are hard to tell, harder to hear or truly witness – "but it's hard to tell the story of this project in the same voice that I had six years ago when I started. When it started, it was raw pain. Now, when I talk, it is more of a story that I have perspective on – not perspective like I'm at a distance, but what I have experienced in doing this project has profoundly changed my own life. Now, I am more at peace."

The first time I met Assaf was at a Halloween party: an oddly prescient setting given how much of our conversation, at least in the beginning, would center on almost unspeakable darkness. After ten minutes of extremely small talk, he suddenly stopped and looked at me rather earnestly. His pause then gave way to a sudden "But enough about all this, pain recognizes pain, and I want to know what happened to you." His quiet sincerity was the only thing keeping his question from being outrageously inappropriate. Rather than finding myself offended, I was intrigued. Who would ask such a question, and why? I realized in retrospect this response must be quite common in Assaf's world; he has made an artistic practice of such inquiries. As a photographer he asks, "How are you?" and actually wants an answer. Sometimes he waits years, but again and again he solicits the deepest possible answer. In doing so, things change.

When we talk about this project, he comes back to the stories of the people that inspired his work and the changes that their lives and their stories have wrought in him, in his work. He usually starts with the story of Sassy, the model who allowed the project to take root. "She passed away two years ago, and she is still leading me to people. She became the key that opened many doors. The relationship was mutually beneficial. For example, in exchange for my support with her rent, she enabled me to use her apartment several times to photograph models who didn't have a home. Her inspirational affect on me was as powerful as mine on her. Maybe she came from a place that was less lucky, but there was no 'who is more and who is less.'"

At times Assaf mentions the death of his father, and the moment in his life when *Scar Tissue* began to take shape again. He'll interrupt himself to assure me that this project existed forever, since the beginning, since the day he pulled a book by Diane Arbus off the shelf in

Art school and realized what kind of work he was drawn to, the work he would do. How he knew right then that it was the pain, the darkness, the suffering that united the stories he wanted to tell with his work. His voice gets softer when he talks about what happened after that realization: his leaving Israel, and coming to the States, leaving everything to get away from that knowing and dumping photography along the way. His voice rises again when he recalls the fifteen years of paralysis that followed, years of guilt for not doing what he knew he had to do. He pauses for a moment before revealing that it was only on the death of his father that the work reemerged, connections began forming, the camera returned, and the *Scar Tissue* project was initiated.

If the work was there from the beginning, to understand it in context we must go back to Assaf's beginning, and a childhood of immense suffering. "This part of my past is important because it has to do with how I was silenced. When you put someone under the water they cannot scream." As we puzzle through how much of his childhood to disclose in these pages, how much of the suffering to detail without it being too much, we come up against the limits of language, of storytelling, to adequately express experience. But the work at hand is in many ways a refracted mirror of this very experience, and disclosure lies at its very heart. And so we return again and again to the bathtub, the freezing water, to holding his breath. To know Assaf is to know that he was raised by an extremely unpredictable and violent mother, a mother whose pain and anger inflicted years of heinous abuse on his body, mind and soul. It is the bathtub that perhaps best tells this story, because she would literally try and drown him daily. What does a child do under such circumstances, how does he survive? "I learned to hold my breath for a very long time" he says softly with a wry, unassuming smile.

The private hell that Assaf experienced began early – before words, before even the possibility of understanding. "What can a one-year-old understand?" he asks aloud when we speak of it. But growth brought with it the knowledge that he was not just a victim of his mother's unbalance, but of the silence kept by the adults around him. "The public realm was her *forté* – she would get even more excited, more crazy." Neighbors in Assaf's desert city lived in close proximity. "She went on rampages daily, many times a day, when she would yell, hit, spank, strike, scream, all in the yard, in the street, in front of everyone. When other kids were playing in the street, if they were playing in front of her house during her siesta she would get up half-dressed, not dressed, and she would come out and yell at them, turn on the lawn sprinkler or even chase the kids with the hose. She seemed to have some fixation with water. . ."

"I was punished all the time. I would be blamed and punished for things I had never done, even crying was a reason to be punished. If my brother or sisters did something, I was punished – it had nothing to do with reality. I told her from a very young age that I had fantasies about having other mothers, I thought it was normal – she told me it was normal to want another mother. I would think about the mothers of my friends, who saw in me this quiet, shy, well-behaved kid. . ." In any conversation with Assaf, there are almost too many stories from childhood to imagine. I wonder aloud how things evolved as he got older, in part because it is difficult to imagine how he survived to become the gentle man who was now speaking. "The first time I drew a boundary with her was when I was about 12 years old. She was chasing me, I can't remember why. I was running and running and she was about to catch me and hit me. For some reason, I turned around and grabbed her hands and said," – he looks at me deeply and intently when he says this – "you're not going to hit me any more." We stop talking for a moment, sitting quietly. Eventually he says, "The yelling never stopped, never, but the physical abuse, at least, stopped then."

In November of 2008, Assaf presented a portfolio of images at the University of California State of the Arts conference. Attended mostly by academics, but with a strong contingent of local artists and community members, Assaf's quiet nature and gentle manner contrasted considerably with the loquaciously analytic crowd. Given the close connection between his personal history and the work at hand, his short reminiscence, a few words on the topic of his own suffering, were both moving and appropriate. The conference facilities were larger than life – cavernous ceilings that somehow dwarfed the enormous stage and video screen behind Assaf's small podium. Lit brightly from above in a darkened room, his low, soft voice sharply amplified, completed the effect: he seemed impossibly small, fragile, and quiet for such a startling message. He said very little, sharing a few words about his background – alluding directly to his abusive upbringing before shyly stepping aside for a series of images from the *Scar Tissue* series unfolding on the giant screen behind him. To the strains of an Israeli lament or prayer, many of the photographs in the current collection illuminated the room for a few moments before fading into the next. Here the size and depth of the work, in contrast to the quiet voice of the artist himself, came loudly into focus.

It is the intimacy in the black and white portraits that made their translation to the big screen so striking. Like the amplification of Assaf's quiet voice, the enormity of the emotional impact of his work was almost overwhelming at this size. But Assaf himself seemed immune to the effect, and literally sprang to life the moment he could engage the audience in dialogue. Not surprisingly, one of the most ardent audience responses was about exploitation. When asked if, given the nature of the photographs and their subjects, the work constituted exploitation of the pain of others, Assaf challenged the assumptions about his role as photographer in this question. He understands his work as a mutual exchange, documenting human connection that went far beyond the images. The true subject of Assaf's photos is both the person, *and* what exists between them. This collaborative approach and deep connection to the souls in each image is perhaps the most nuanced element the body of work shares. In other words, what unites all the photographs beyond printing technique, film stock and the photographer's eye is the atmosphere created at the moment of their capture. Not one of setting or objects, but of trust, vulnerability and openness. This can't be staged, or rushed, or achieved opportunistically. The images capture years of intense interaction, mutual vulnerability, and shared risk.

"How do you build trust with someone who has so little ability to trust? It is a huge issue. I, personally, cannot betray them because they've already been so betrayed." In the end, Assaf's story is only one of the stories here. There is no way to give words to all the experiences behind the eyes captured in these pages, but Sassy embodies much of their spirit – and no erfully shaped the work from early in the process. When Assaf met "Sassy" she was working as a submissive in one of the professional BDSM houses in Los Angeles, and just released from prison. "She was in the custody of her (BDSM) master during her parole, so to talk to me she had to ask permission from her master first. I felt she didn't trust me, that like many of us, including myself, her ability to trust was severely damaged in childhood." The first moment he saw her tells the story – a female dom responded to Assaf's mentioning the title *Scar Tissue* by offering that she had "someone with a good scar for you," before bellowing "Sassy! Come Here! Show him your scar!!" Sassy emerged quickly from a back room and complied, lifting her worn T-shir to a complete stranger without question or objection. Assaf asked before he left that day if she might be interested in modeling for his project, and she agreed.

At first the progress was slow. "We met several weeks later, and she told me her whole story. But she told me before we met very specifically that she wasn't going to cry. She told me about her surgery, her valve replacement. In prison she was given a physical, and they found out she needed a valve replacement in her heart because of her years of heroin addiction. So she went through this surgery, and spent time in prison. When I met her it was a short time after she was released. We started to work, and we photographed, she opened up and cried a lot. In her search to finally find someone who would see, accept and love her she was willing to do anything, almost without boundaries. Then we didn't see each other for about ten days, but we arranged for another meeting. When we met again she told me that after the photography session she hadn't stopped crying for the whole time we were apart. She told me that it was the first time she felt like someone could hear and understand her. We connected as two people in a powerful spiritual way. We shared stories. She started calling me a lot for advice. Then she threw a birthday party at her new place for her friend Sofya, and she invited me. The party was a door to the BDSM community, because most of the people there were from the scene, and we drove all the way to Passive Arts Studios (a professional dungeon/club) for a suspension party – the birthday girl got suspended with hooks."

"Soon Sassy became really identified with *Scar Tissue* as a project. She would find other folks, other models, so that they could also go through this process. Not for me, but for them. Eventually I helped her to move to her own apartment. She and her girlfriend rented an apartment for the first time in her life. All the time through our relationship she tried to get out of this life, to become a "normal person" – she found a job at Whole Foods and kept that job for the rest of her life. This incredible woman started at the very bottom of everything, and through all this effort she wanted to become something, to have a "normal" life. She wanted to give birth to a "normal" child. Her dream to give birth did come true, but sadly, Sassy didn't live to see her child.

Sassy's own words for this project, which she put on paper shortly before she died, reveal the depths from which she emerged, and the many ghosts from her past still clinging. The childlike quality of her prose at striking odds with the darkness of her tale:

> It seems strange to me to sit here and put 'me' on paper. I feel as if I will be open, vulnerable to ridicule and a let down to many.

I grew up without a lot of things in my life, being molested when I was 11 or 12, Dad being in prison all my younger years, then me having to grow up so quickly I feel as if I missed a lot.

During the periods of me becoming a teenager I went through many changes and by the age of 16 I had a little boy whose name was Jack Kenneth Webb III. After two shor months he passed away from Meningitis. I was devastated. . . I got caught up being sad depressed, and drunk, and smoked some [crack cocaine] with my boyfriends to connec Things just overlapped and before I knew what happened I was stuck in the circle o crack-cocaine, pimps, and prostitution. It became a form of survival; after some tim I started to hang with a lot of people who were also doing heroin. Never did I think would venture down that route. Heroin became my 'everything.' I did it for six years an also gained Hep C from it. By the end of my using I had already been arrested 80 times many under the influences, with paraphernalia, prostitution, and drug possessions; I ha been beat up, had pimps put my family through hell and all around hated everything and everybody.

Assaf reveals even more of her difficult story, having been profoundly touched by Sassy's xperiences. "She told me that when she was 13 she left home, and within a few years wa loing drugs and prostitution. She told me she lost another child – this one murdered by the hild's father. She also told me that the one child who is still alive was taken away from he nd raised by brutal uncles more interested in his social security check. Finally, when she hac ler fourth child, it killed her." But this is the part of Sassy's tale that Assaf rarely shares – h s far more enthusiastic about how she was in the process of turning her life around. Sh aised herself up from these circumstances, left abusive relationships, got off of drugs an got a job. She got her driver's license a few months before she passed away, and was looking orward to having another child – this time being the mother she'd always wanted to be. He ife was in the process of transformation, and it was this transformation that most excited an nspired Assaf about their work together, their friendship, and Sassy's powerful influence o he project. It is this transformation that Assaf documented in their work together.

Ultimately, it is transformation that lies at the heart of the work at hand, stretching back o Assaf's earliest relationship to photography. "In the subconscious of a child, my subcon scious, I dealt with a person who had no sense of reality, this is why I wasn't drawn to paint ng, it doesn't document reality, photography documents reality." Assaf sometimes digresse when he talks about his family to discuss how he was drawn into photography – the two ar ntegrally linked. "Since I remember I got punished for things that I didn't do. She [Assaf's nother] was creating her own reality, and I was punished for disagreeing with her percep ion of reality. I talked to her recently and she doesn't remember the bathtub or anything This was my issue always, my own self-doubt. I was punished for seeing reality in a differen way than she did. Sometimes as I walked into the house I would be dragged into the bath ub for a "treatment." I didn't know why. I just walked in to all this violence, with very low yelling and screaming by a very loud person – and she has no recollection of this, *she doesn't remember.* My father on the other hand had his Nikormat, a camera that Nikon made. Since I remember him he had this camera and he used to take pictures all over the place all the time as a very enthusiastic amateur. What I remember is Kodachrome, because they came in a special package and you had to send them away to America. They would come back after a month. From the time I was a little kid I remember we would have these slide shows. We would spend all this time looking at these cartridges of where he traveled, his work, family travels. They were beautiful; the colors were beautiful. He gave me the idea that he was there because he had taken a picture – there was a flower there because he took the picture. I got this idea that I wanted a camera and I got one, a little plastic camera, an Agfa Isopac. It had these 35mm cartridges with square frames. The camera had a fixed focus, and a scratchy lens. But I started to take pictures, and I would take them in all the time to get them developed. Eventually, slowly, slowly he gave me his old Contax, and I felt like I had gotten something really special from my Dad. My favorite subjects were cats and poor men. Even then I was attracted to people, but always to the sad people, the beggars and homeless guys. I would take pictures of cats because I loved them so much, and family. But it was a hobby, nothing more. Today looking back I see that, like my father, taking pictures was my way of seeing reality, of proving that I was there, that something happened. I wanted proof. In my family we keep thinking, "maybe I was wrong, maybe what I think wasn't right." But if there is one photograph, it is there, you can't argue with that. You can't take a picture of something that doesn't exist."

"I took pictures on high school trips, but when I went into military service, photography was just a hobby. I was oriented like the rest of the family to go study engineering or math or something. Then my sister came with this ad for art school, the department of photography was advertising for students. On a Friday she read it to me, and I knew it was difficult to get accepted to this art academy, but spontaneously I was inspired to put in an application and the rest is history." It was there that he met the visionary newspaper editor who changed the concept of journalism in Israel, bringing in the idea that the photograph was as important as the essay. "During a workshop [with this editor], he approached me and said "Come work for me! I'll open any door for you." For many years I worked almost constantly for magazines and didn't realize how burnt out I was. I wouldn't let them choose the photographs for me – I didn't hand them contact sheets, I handed them prints, and almost never did I allow them to be cropped. I didn't realize how consumed I was because this was my life. Photographing, developing, printing, photographing, developing, etc. I didn't have much time for myself. Instead of dealing with my own pain, I was dealing with my pain through others. In a very empathic, well, it's beyond empathic – I identified with them. I craved going to those places. Why was it my obsession to go to the pain, to the outskirts, where there was the most pain? It was a process that I was not in touch with."

But it wasn't until he ventured to America, at the suggestion to a friend, that he recognized something important. "For the first time I was away, it was the first time I felt like I was in a certain emotional spot in my life where I needed to be away. It wasn't the most exciting trip, to say the least, but the break was the first time in my life I was just in a different emotional space. I postponed my return again and again. After a few months, I found myself owning a business, a carpet cleaning business. I ended up in the Fresno/Bakersfield area." Assaf quickly adds that it was the first time he was really away from his mother, too, despite having traveled much in the past. "When I was a student, it was a hard time to get rid of her – when I was in America, it was the first time I was away from her voice. She was sad that her son could leave Israel, but this is the first time I took a break. I started breathing."

"For a long time I didn't have the emotional space to do my photography. Every time I wanted to take a step toward the project, I found all the energy going out of me. The stuff was cooking for 12 years, but I was prevented from realizing it by the fear, the fear blocked me." This was in part due to his family situation. "It wasn't just my father dying that triggered my project, it was coming back to Hawaii [where Assaf's family had a home at the time]. I came back from spending a week burying my father surrounded by the experience of his death and all the family stuff it opened up. . ." He mentions the conflicts that had simmered for years in his family that erupted after his father's death. Assaf's voice trails off a bit at this point, as if the pain in these memories is still very fresh. After a few moments, he continues more softly, more controlled. "I came back home to my family in Hawaii, and my wife could only say, "you were partying in Israel while I had to be alone!" I tried to talk about this with her for several years more, but at the same time I realized that I was being used, I was invisible. This opened me up and freed me up, even though it was painful. It probably accelerated the divorce. She knew *Scar Tissue* was what I wanted to do the whole time, but I couldn't."

So we return to the work at hand, the work that is at once spontaneous and years in the making. The intuitive, interactive process of the photography extends deep into the selection of work for the current collection. "First is how I feel, it's not rational. Even when I select for the book the process is very fast, very intuitive. I don't plan. When I start I have a vague idea, and then I start playing. Memory has a powerful organizing effect on the work, what touches me, has to be an expression of emotion or pain – it must be something that I can see." This dance of memory, play, emotion and connection has its own unique aspects. "[It is] following the flow of the energy. I'm always changing. . . The intuitive process means that things might change – but I select and I don't look back. It is not an analytic process." Thus even the order, grouping and presentation of the work here is spontaneous, intuitive, and emotional. Felt rather than conceived intellectually. *Scar Tissue* required a radical relinquishing of control through meaningful collaboration at all levels from conception through execution. But this is not an incidental artifact of Assaf's working methodology, rather it is a central, and intensely cultivated, characteristic of the artist's person. *Scar Tissue* becomes a multi-layered collection under such circumstances: representing at once many visions and one, thousands of experiences and the work of a single artist, a constantly evolving process illuminated and fixed for a moment in these pages. But that, too, is essential. "The book is more about the message that we all have prejudices that need to be transformed and healed because ultimately we are all connected." This message will continue to deepen, trouble, and challenge the viewer, as the artist himself undoubtedly will.

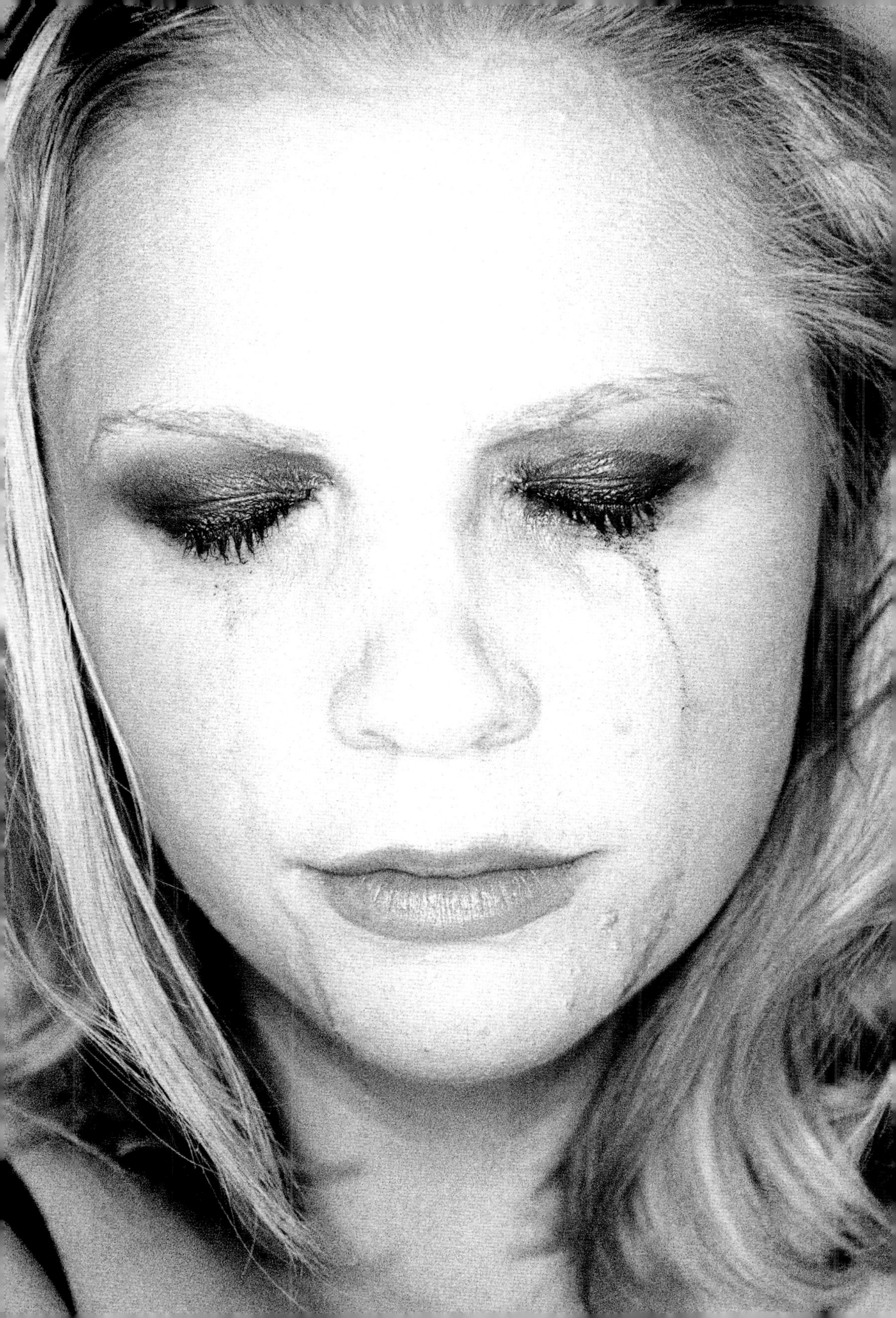

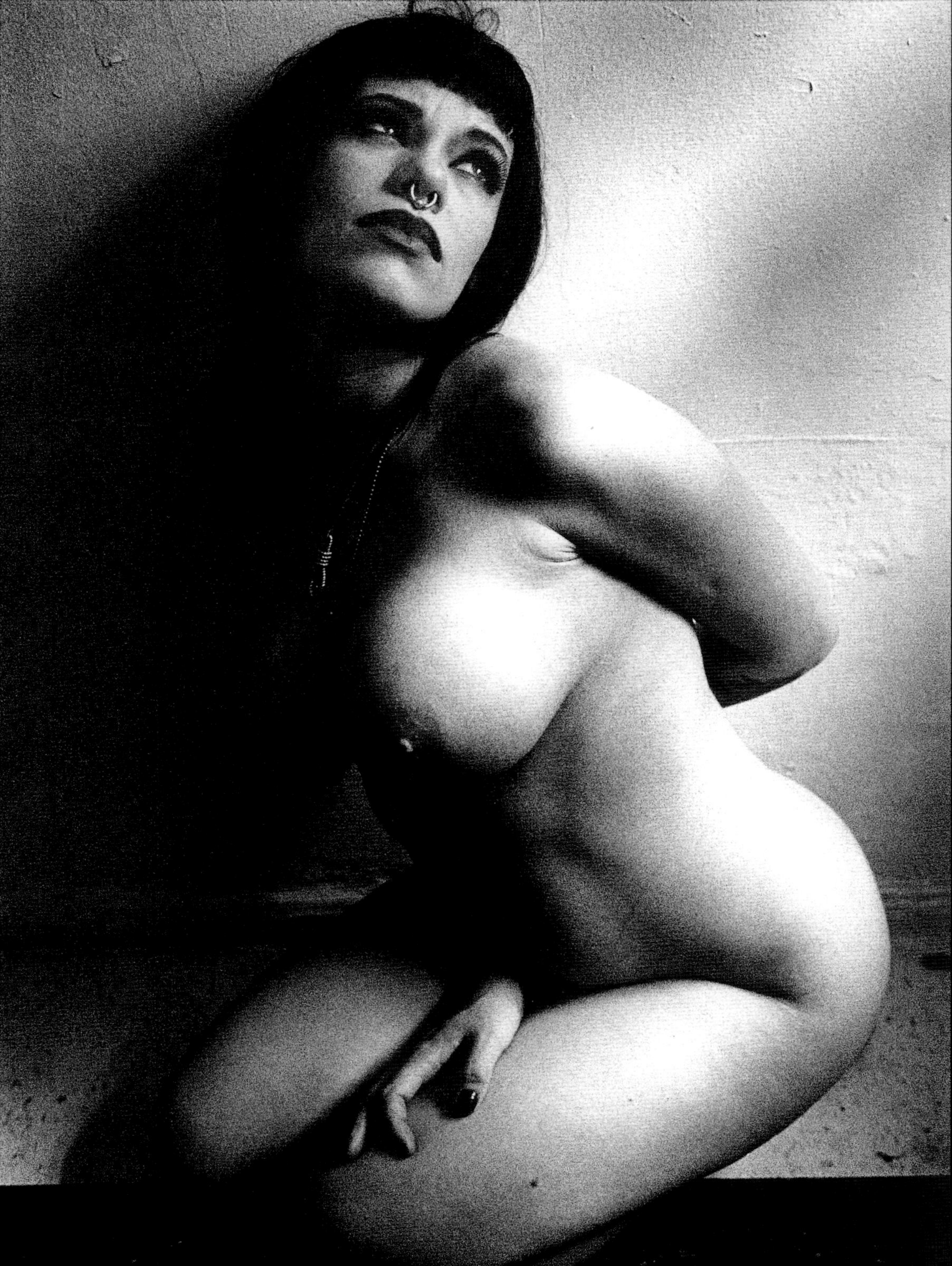

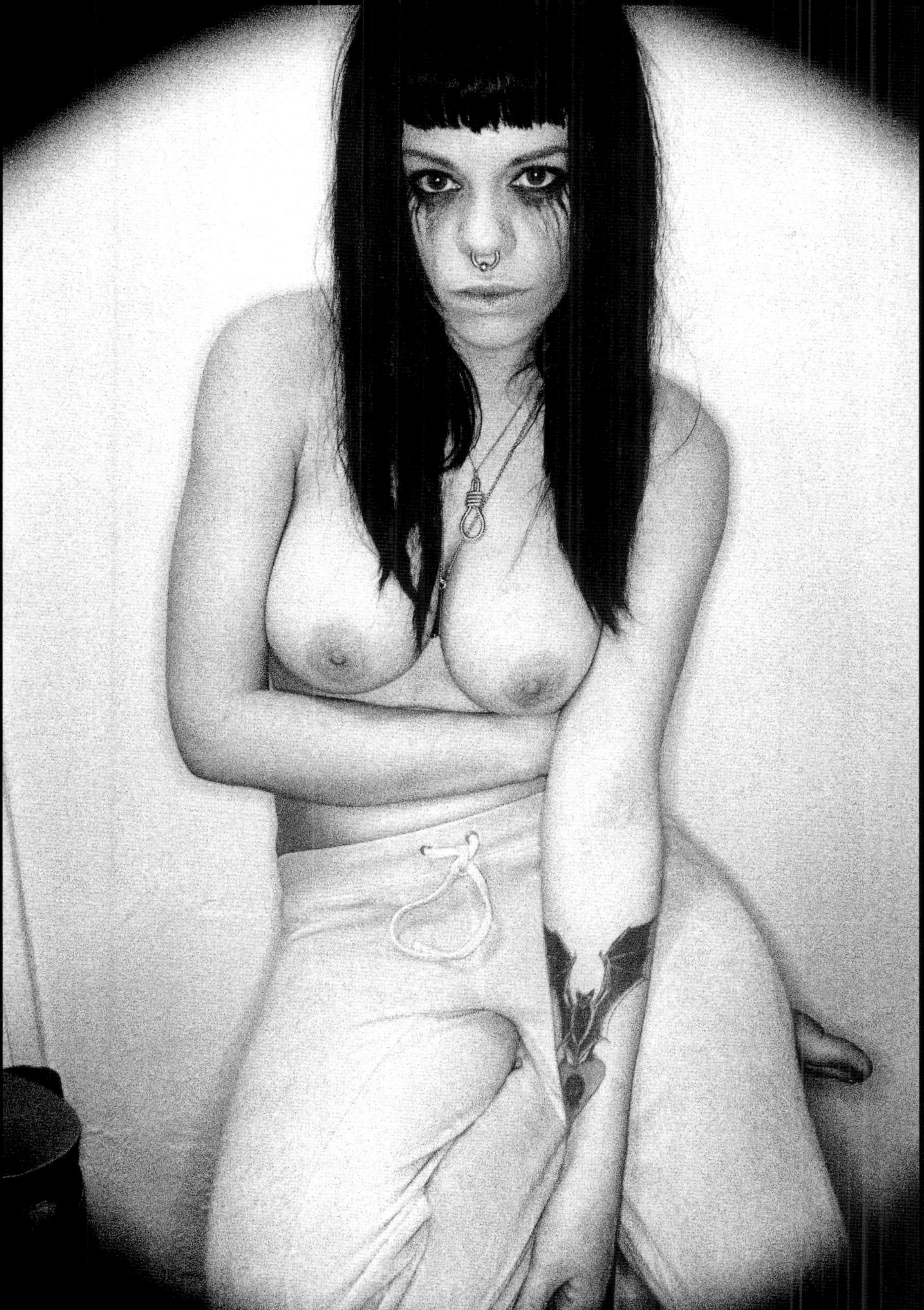

Gia Paloma

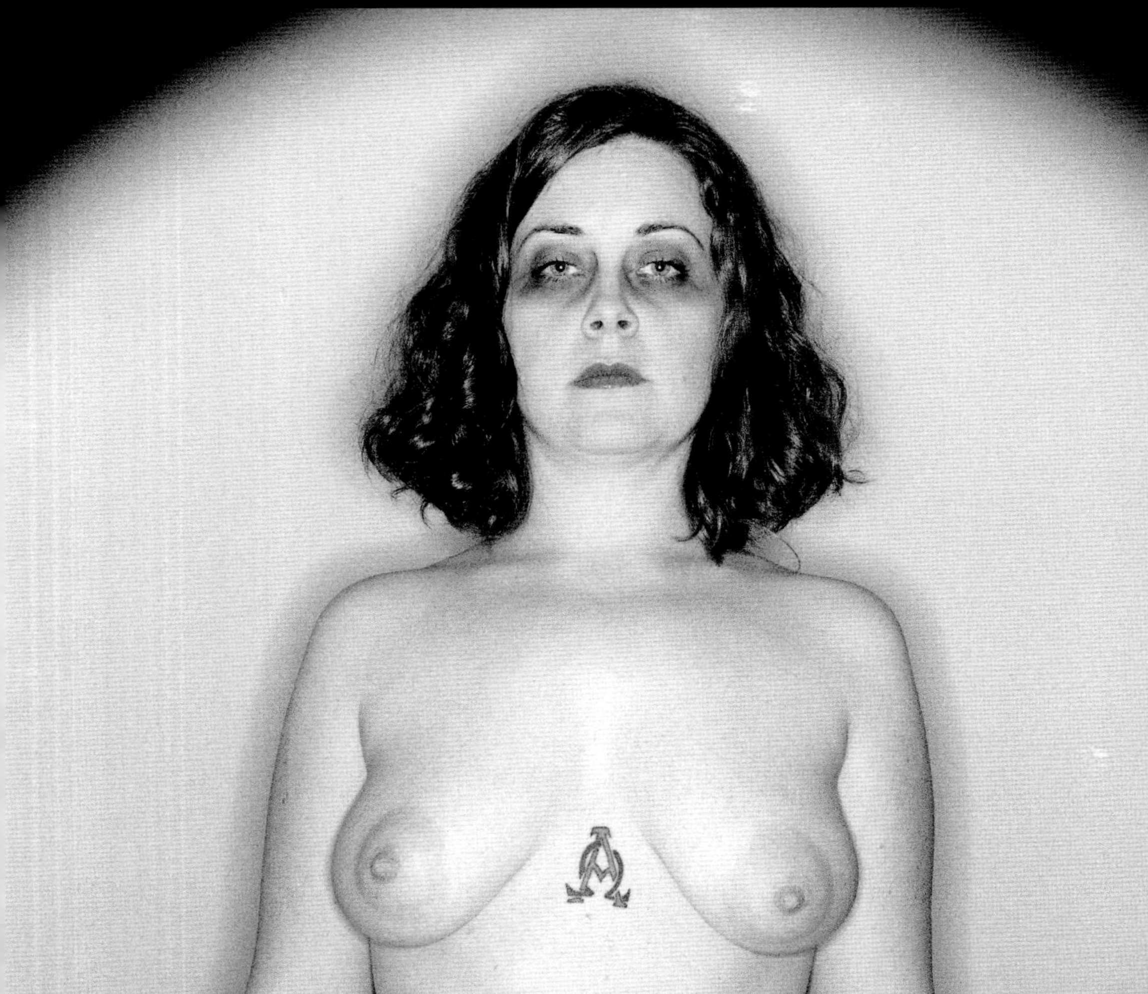

Angela

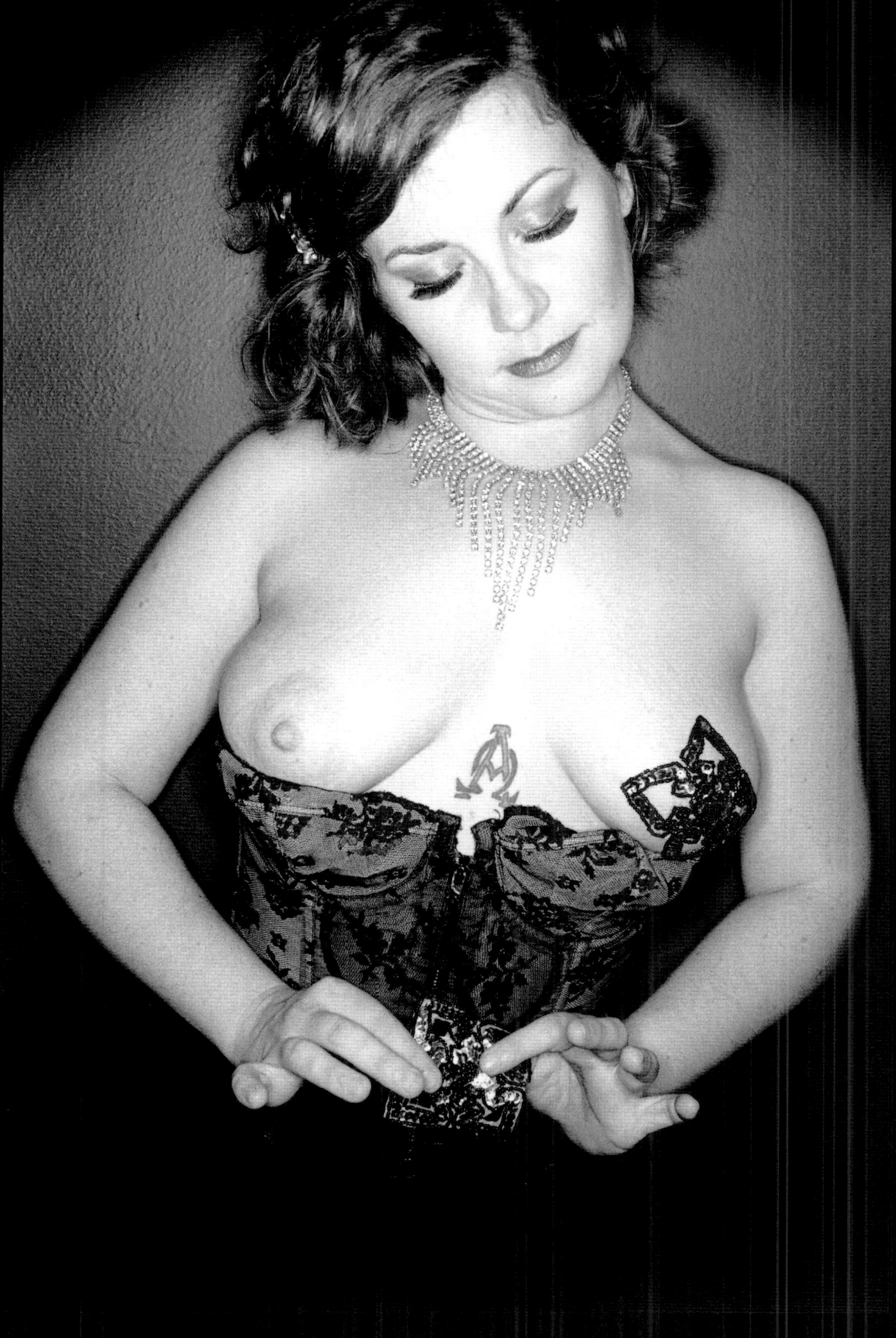

Angela

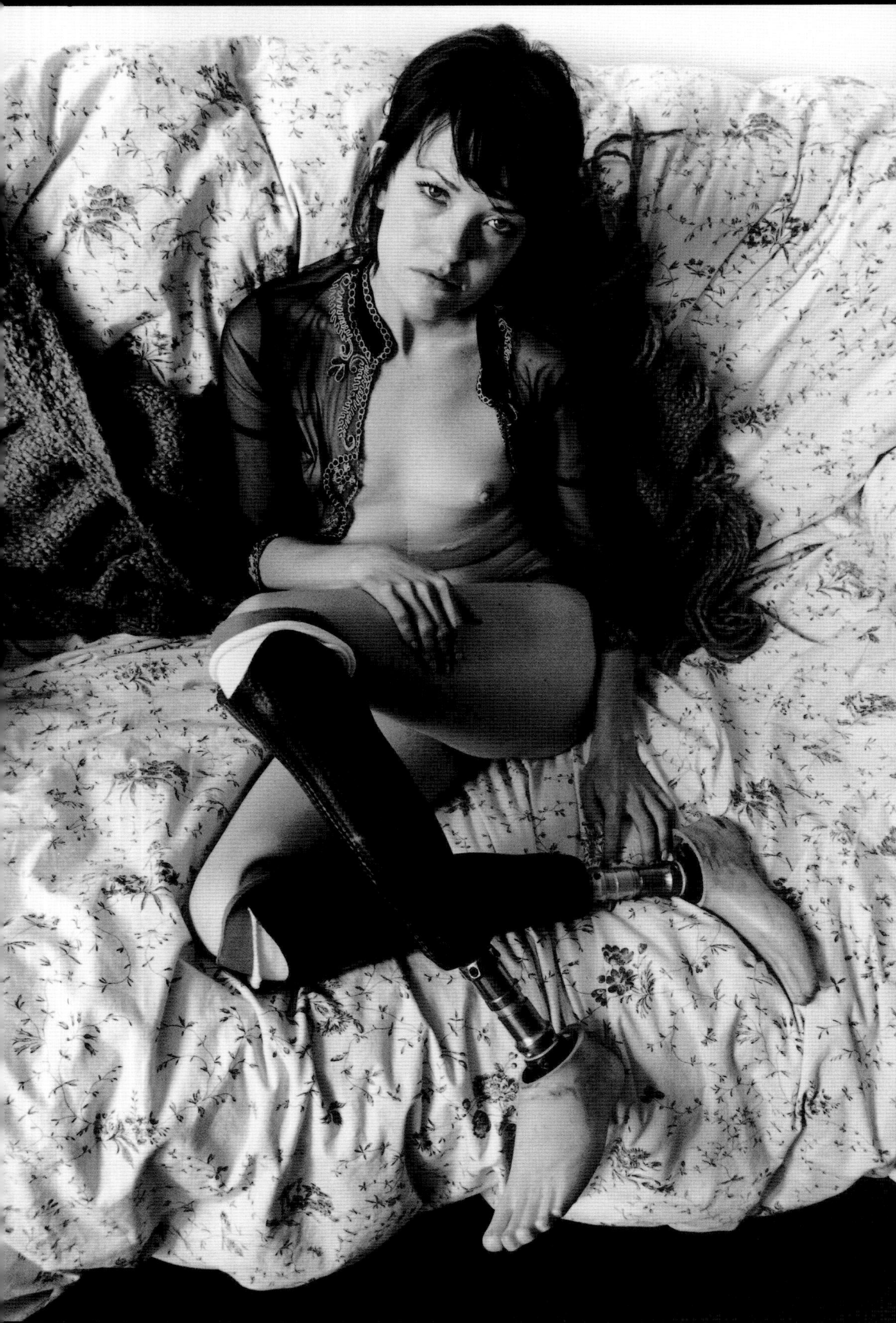

Amy

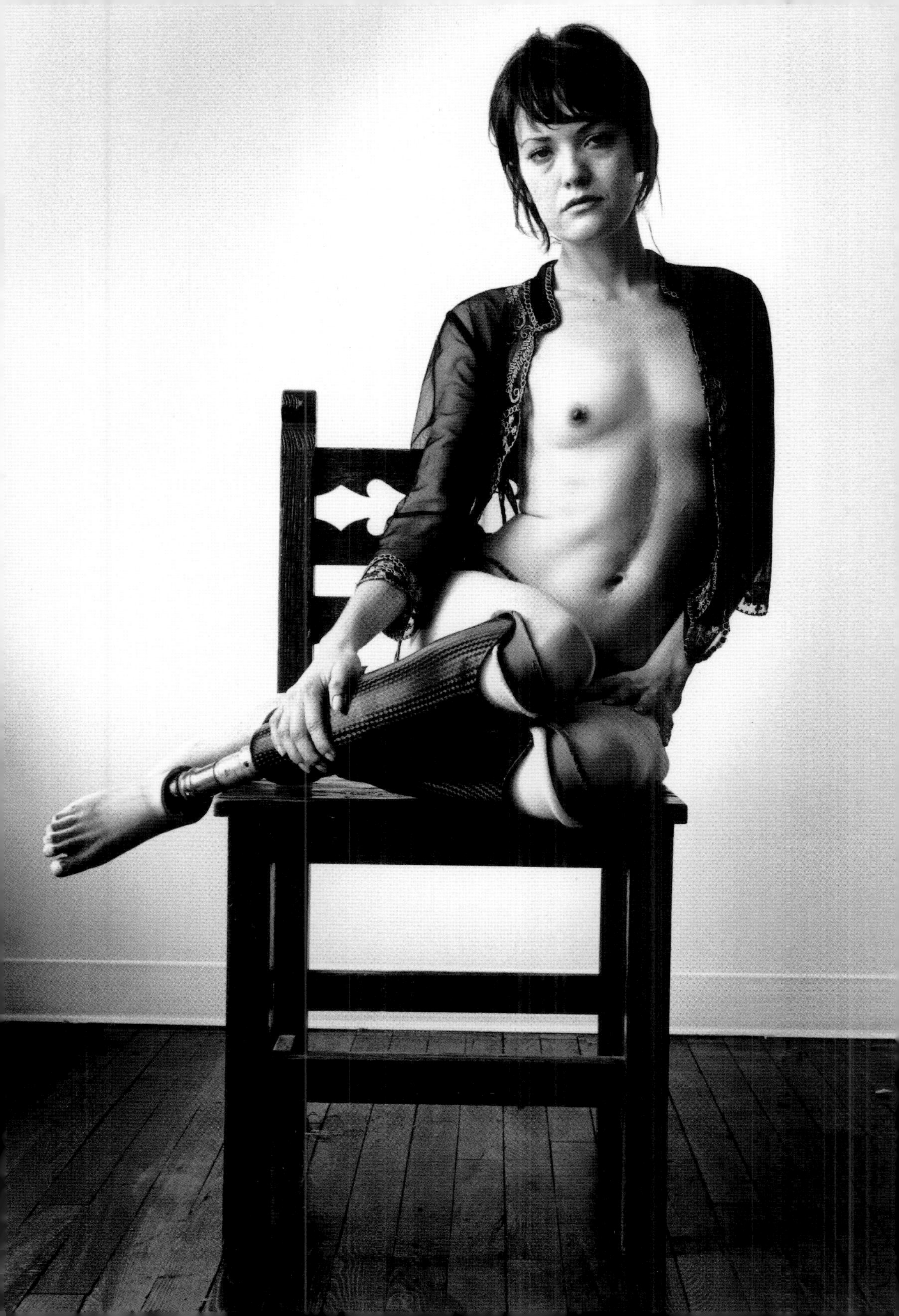

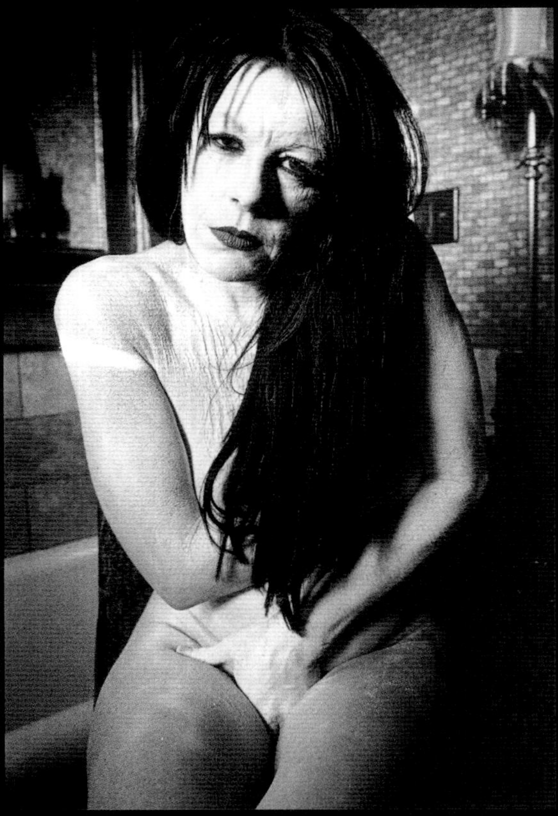
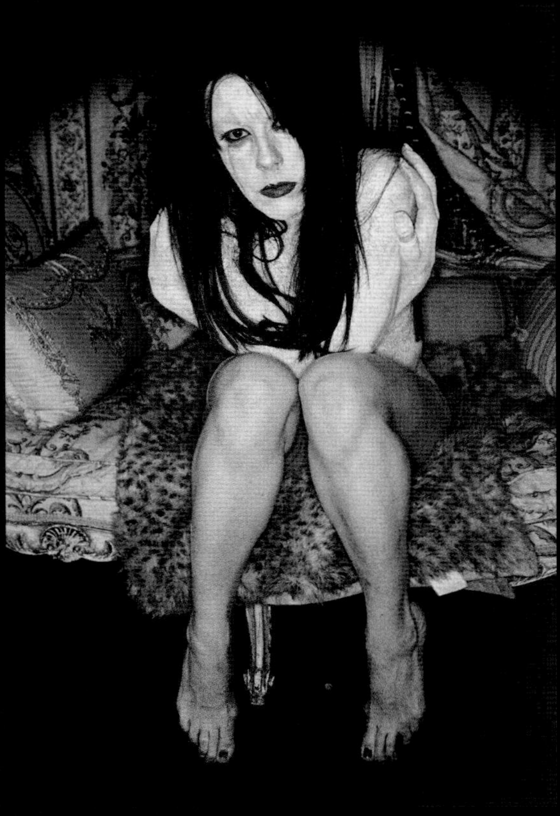
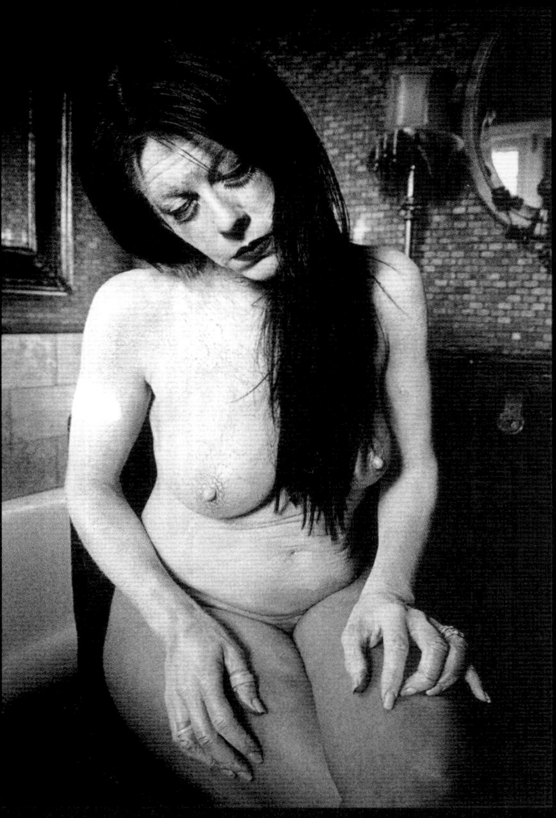
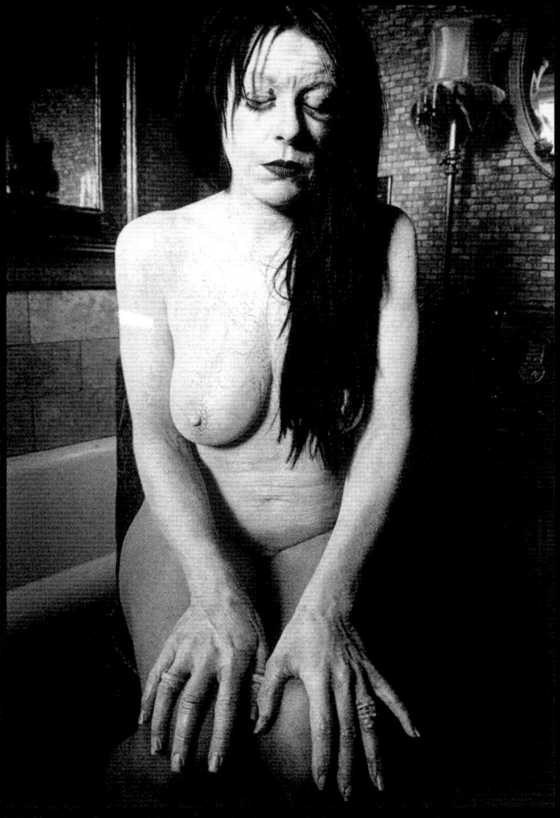

Tiffany

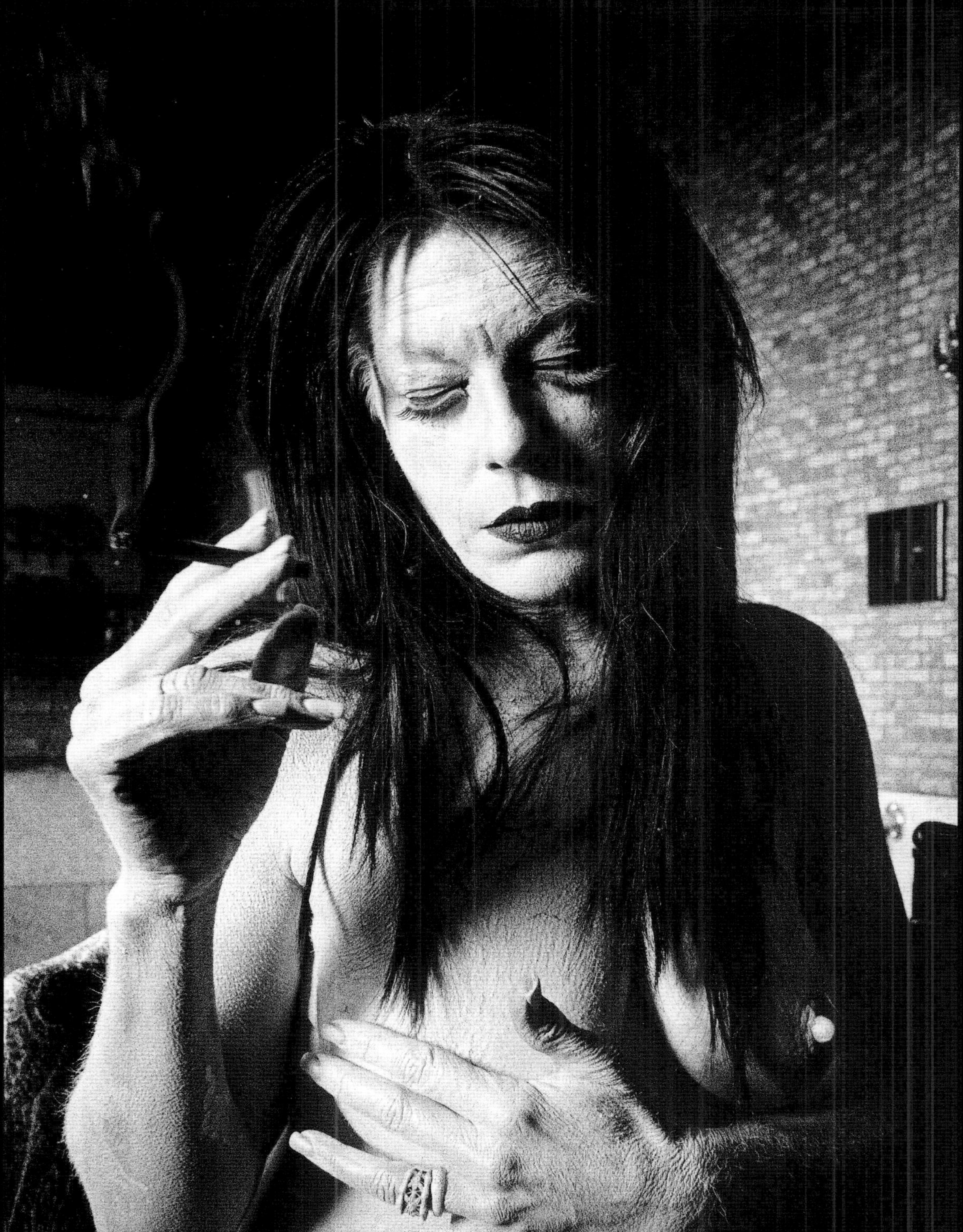

Tiffany

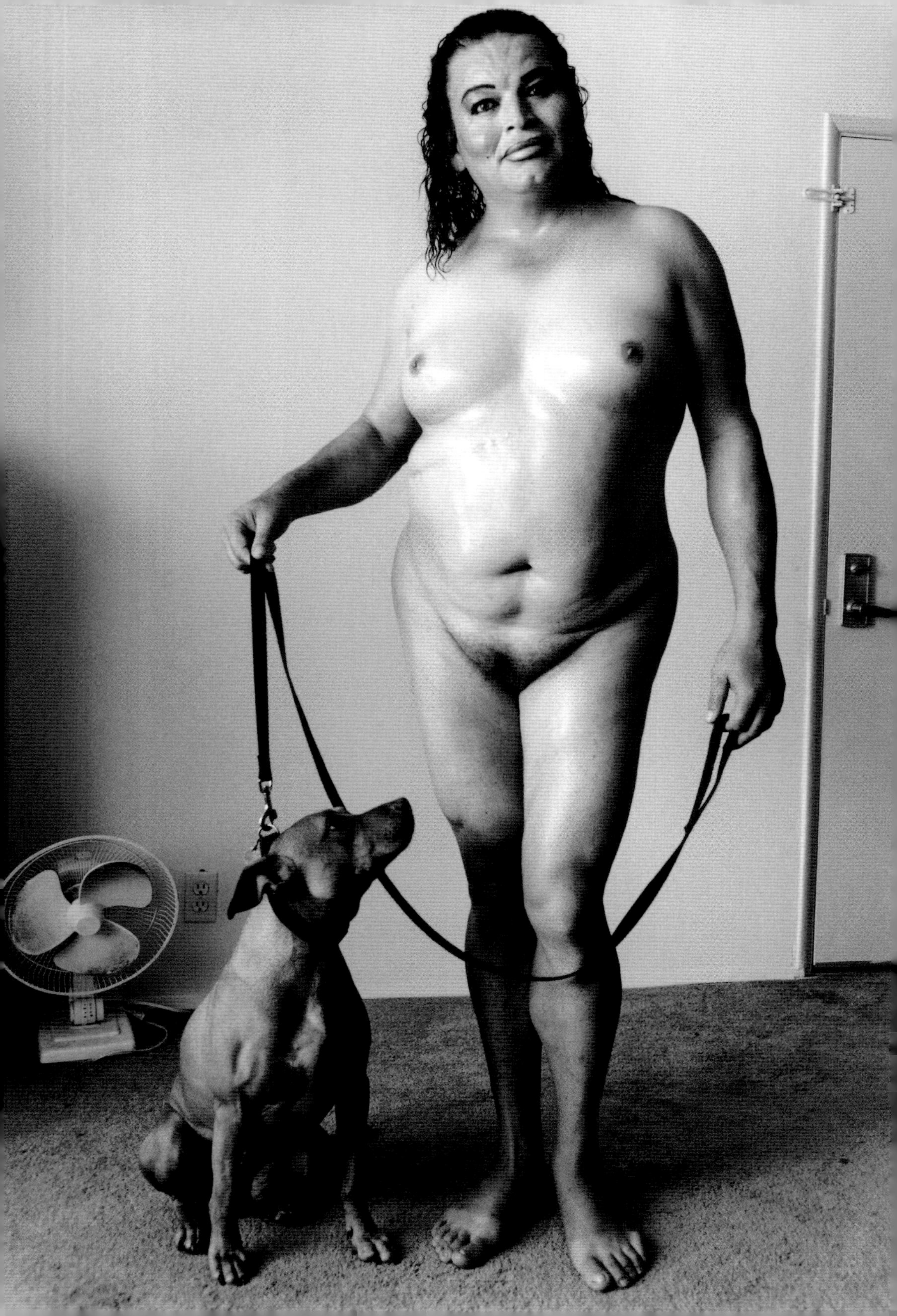

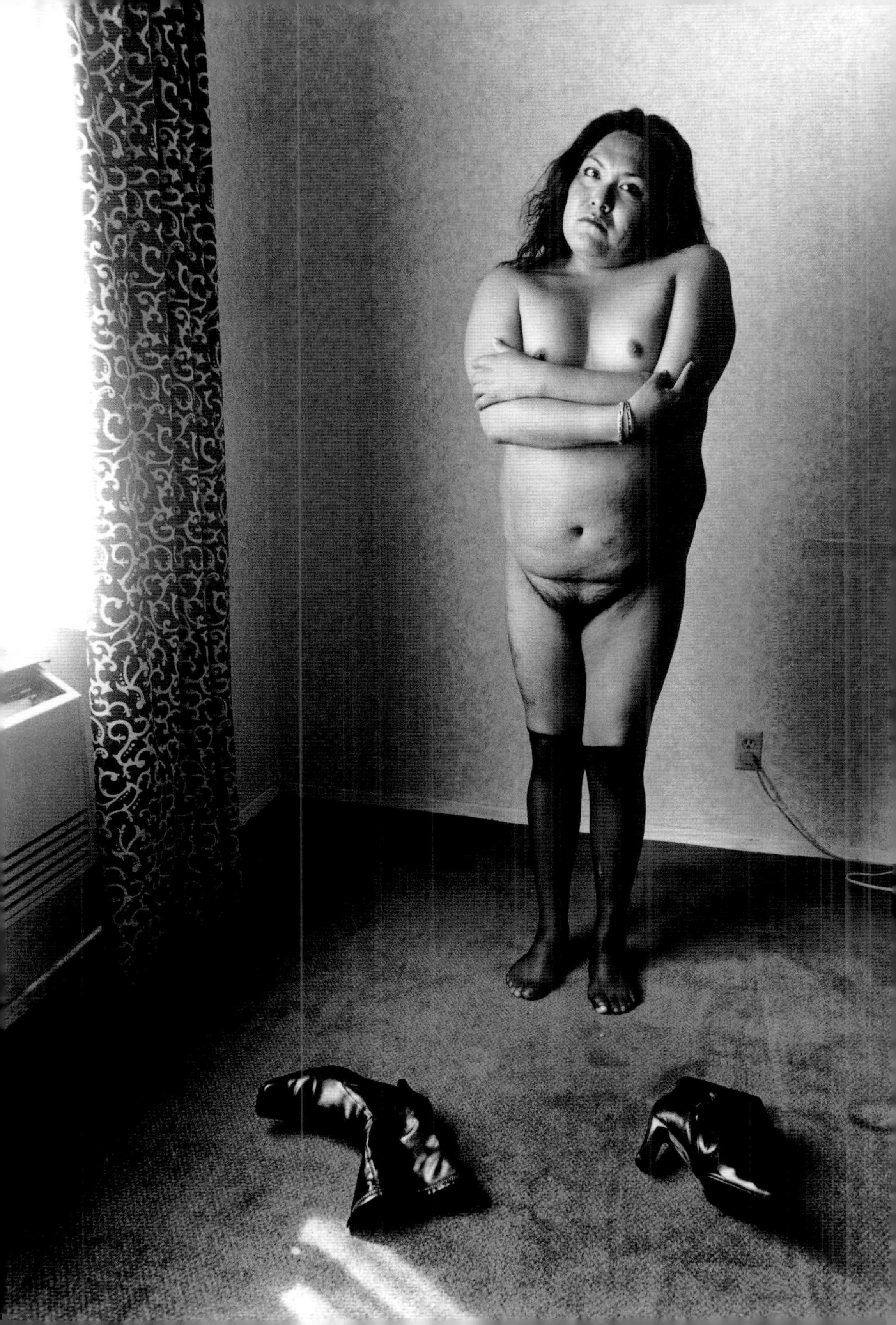

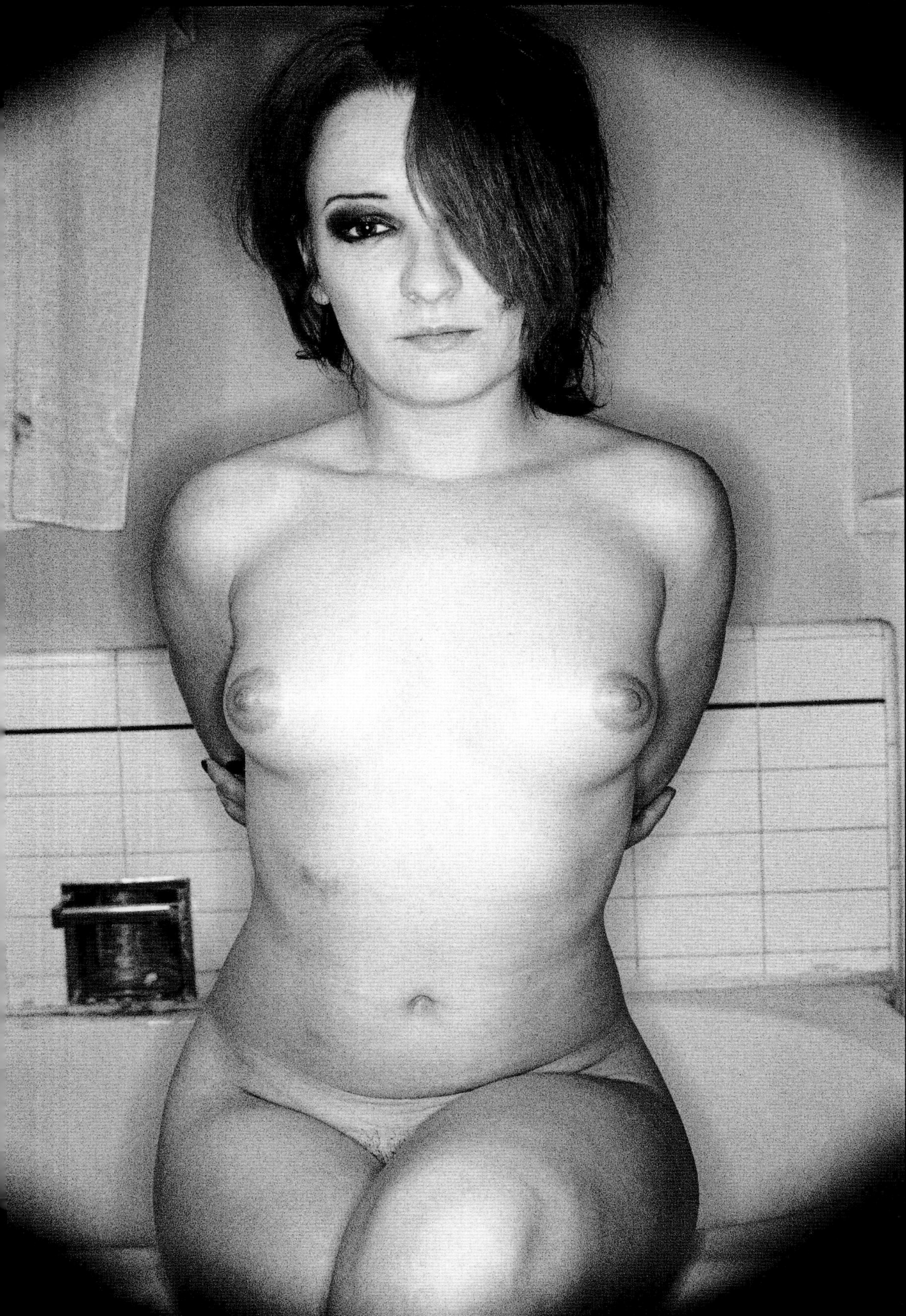

Brandy

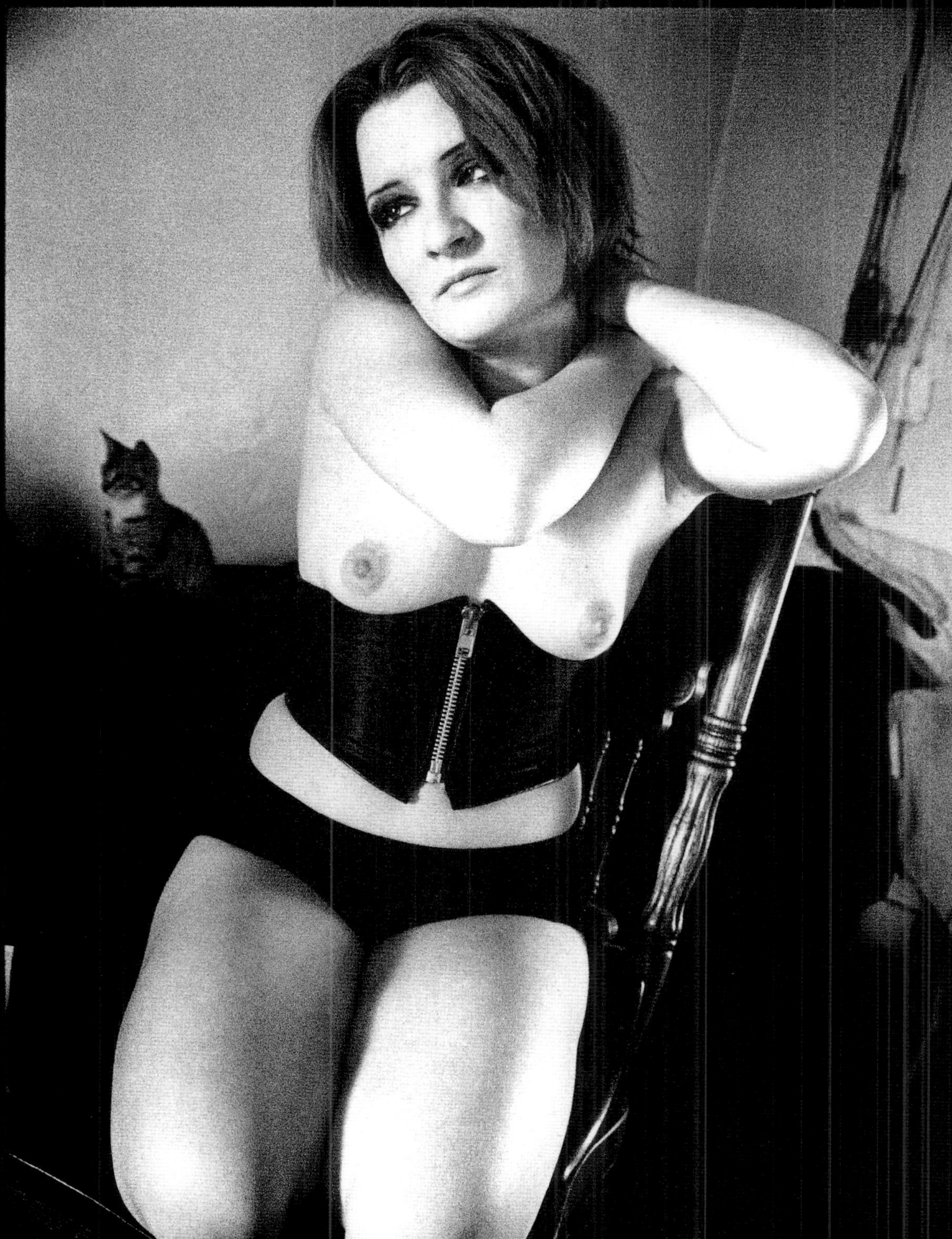

Brandy

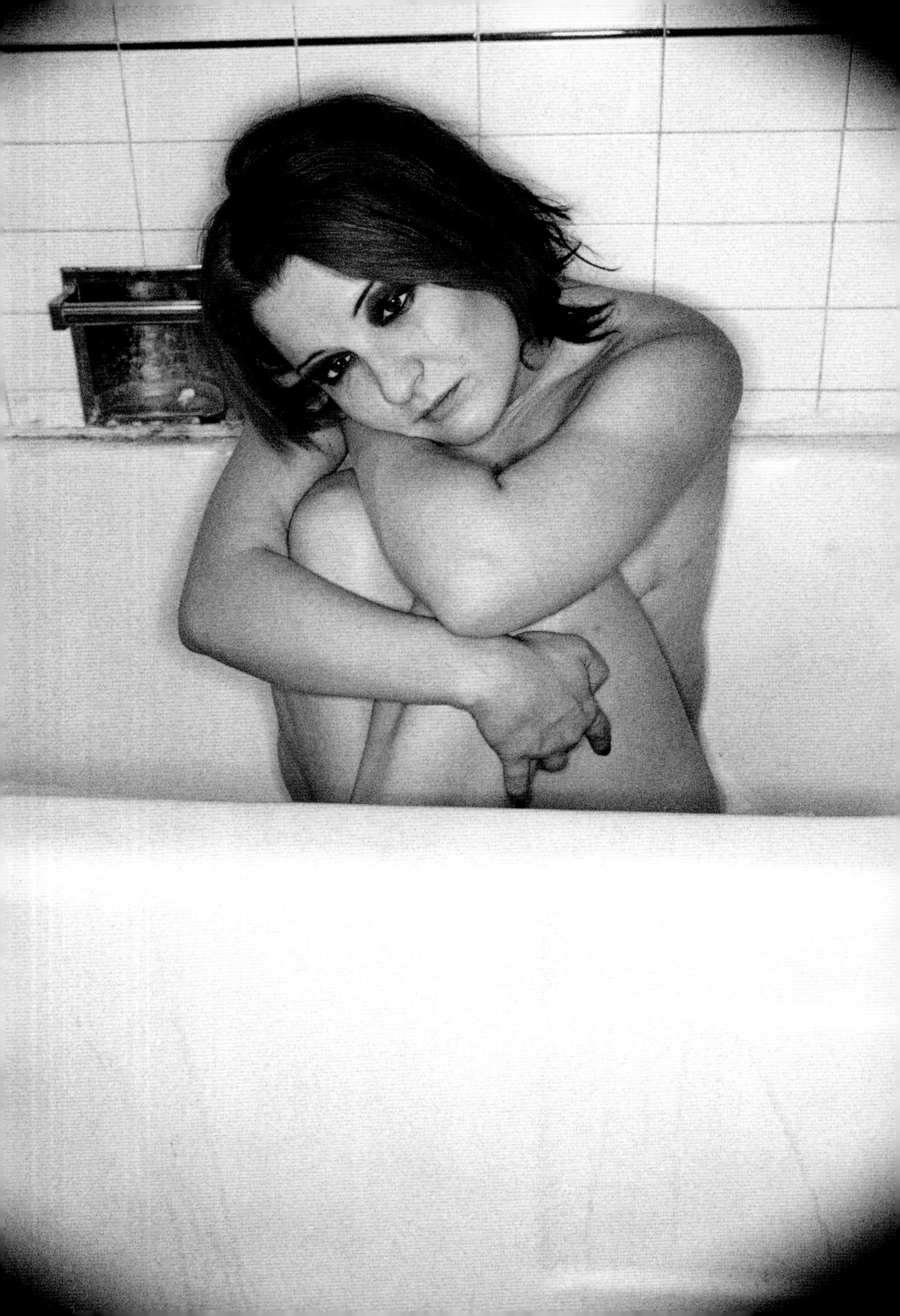

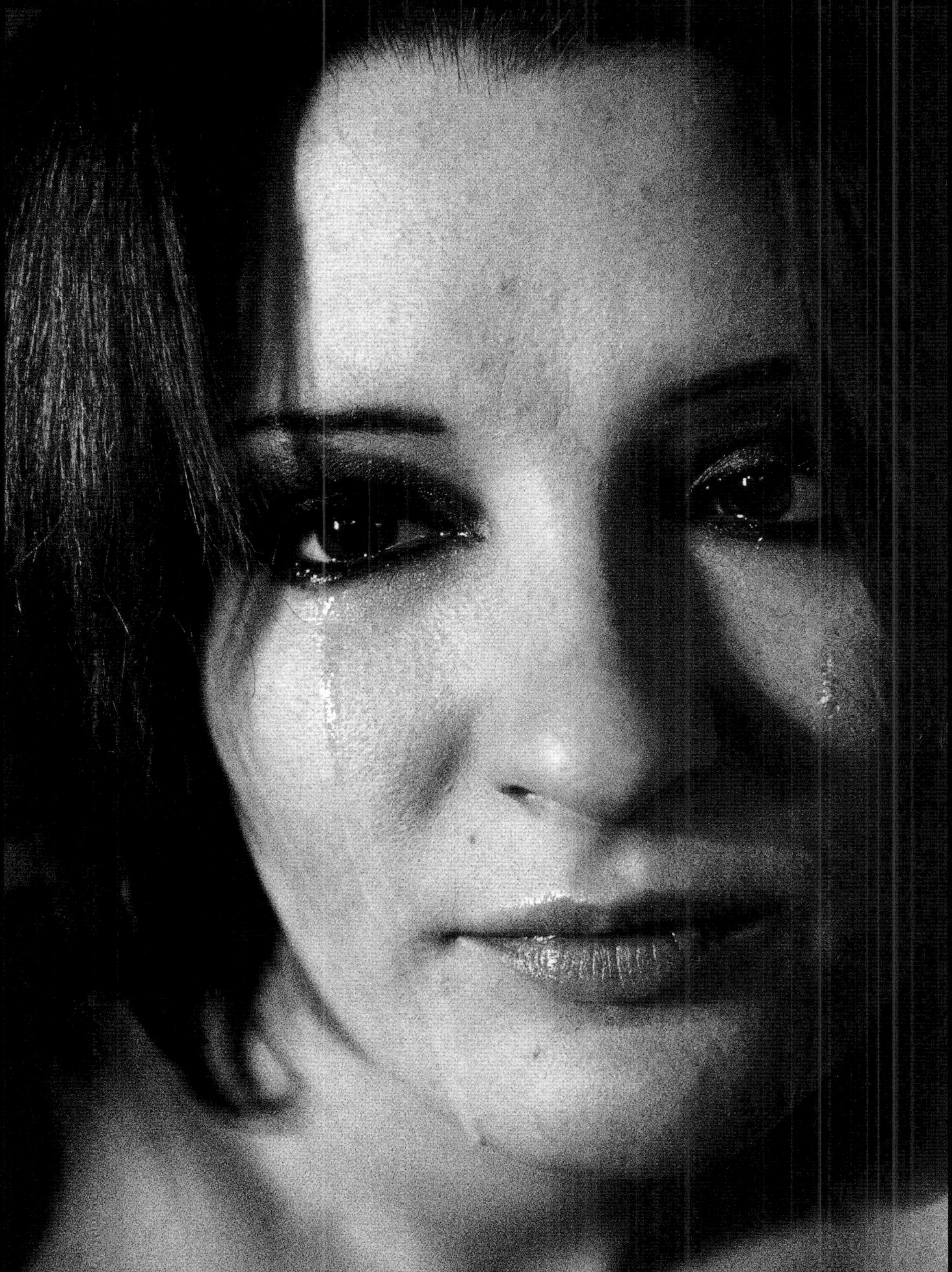

Brandy

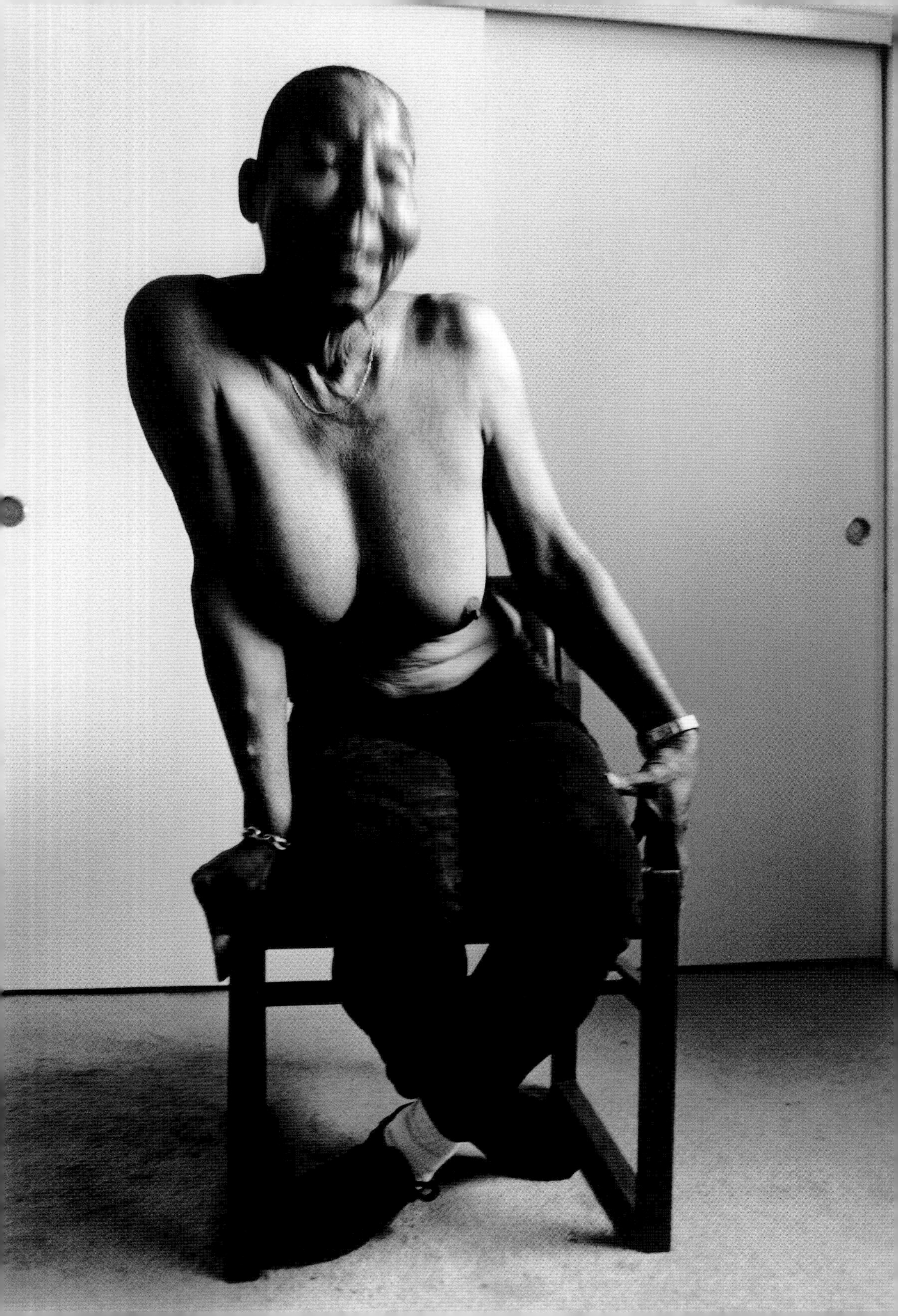

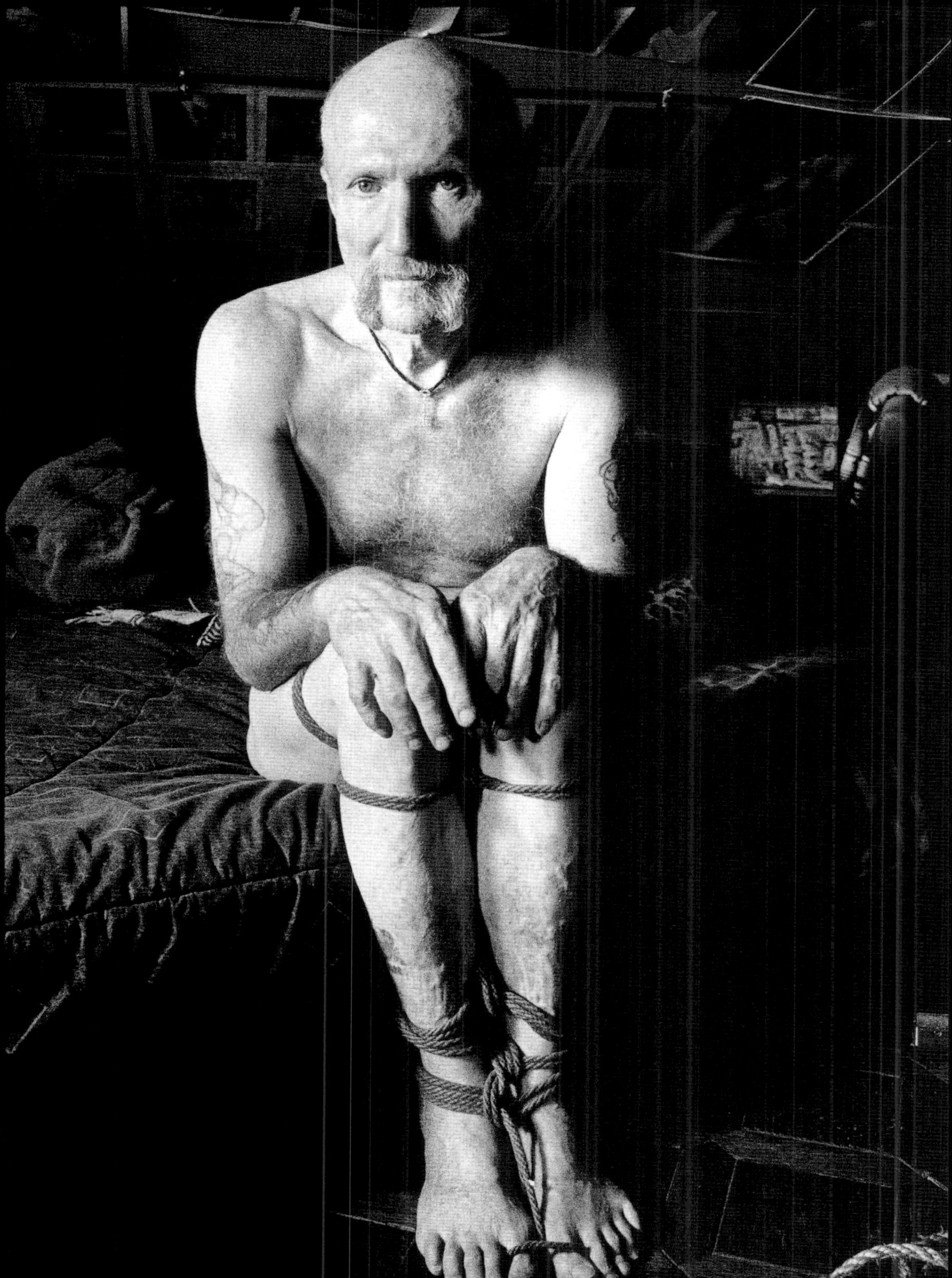

Charley B.

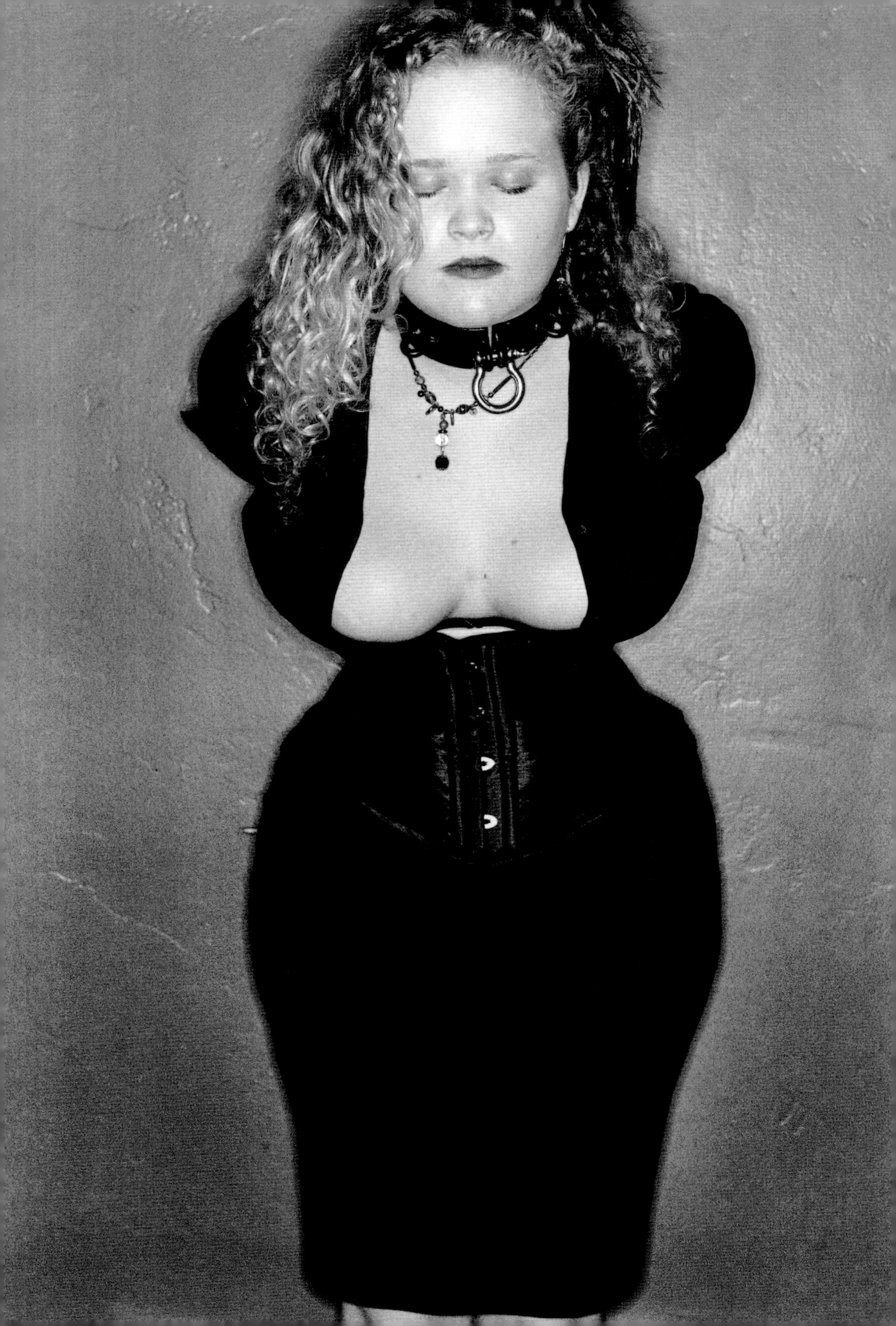

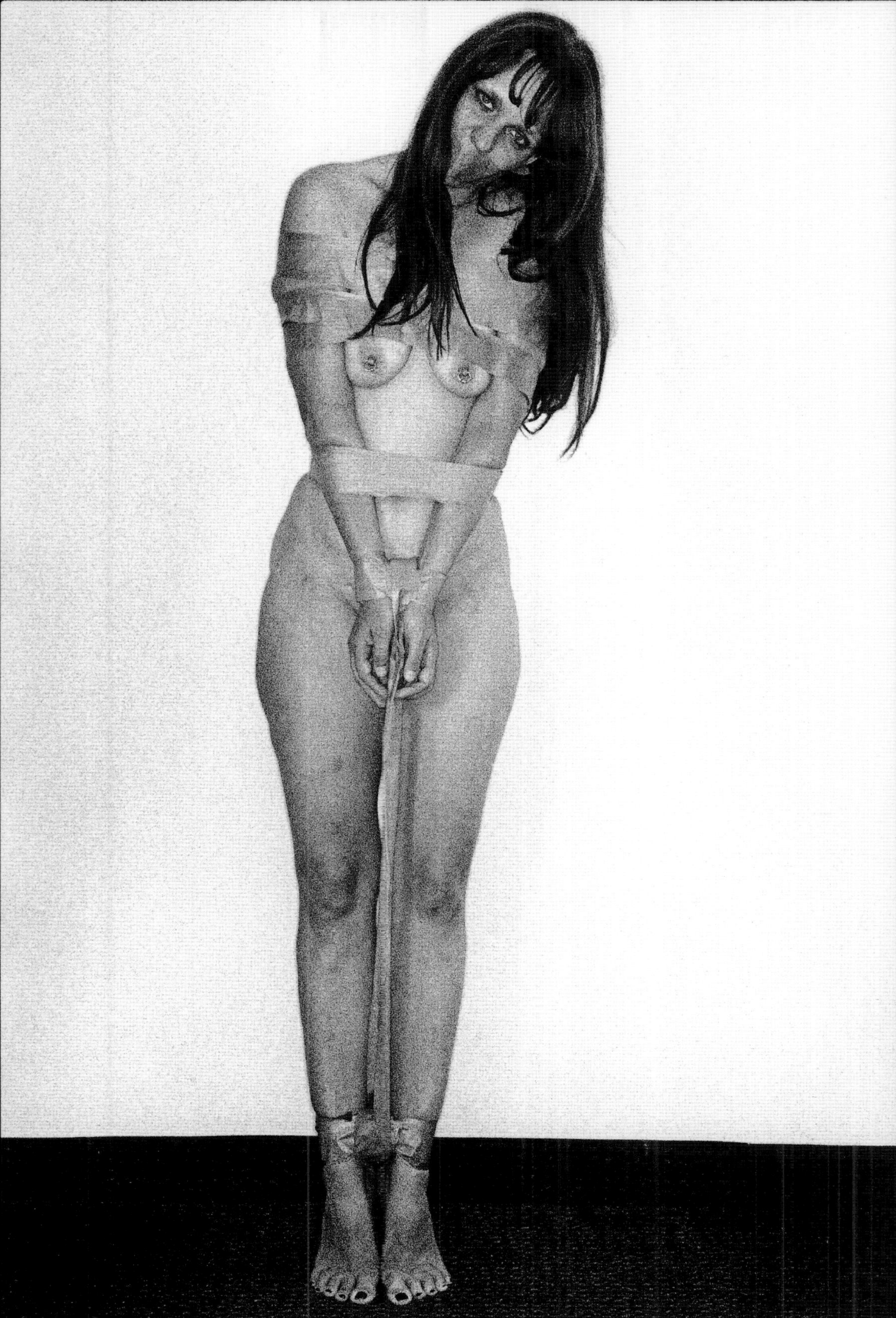

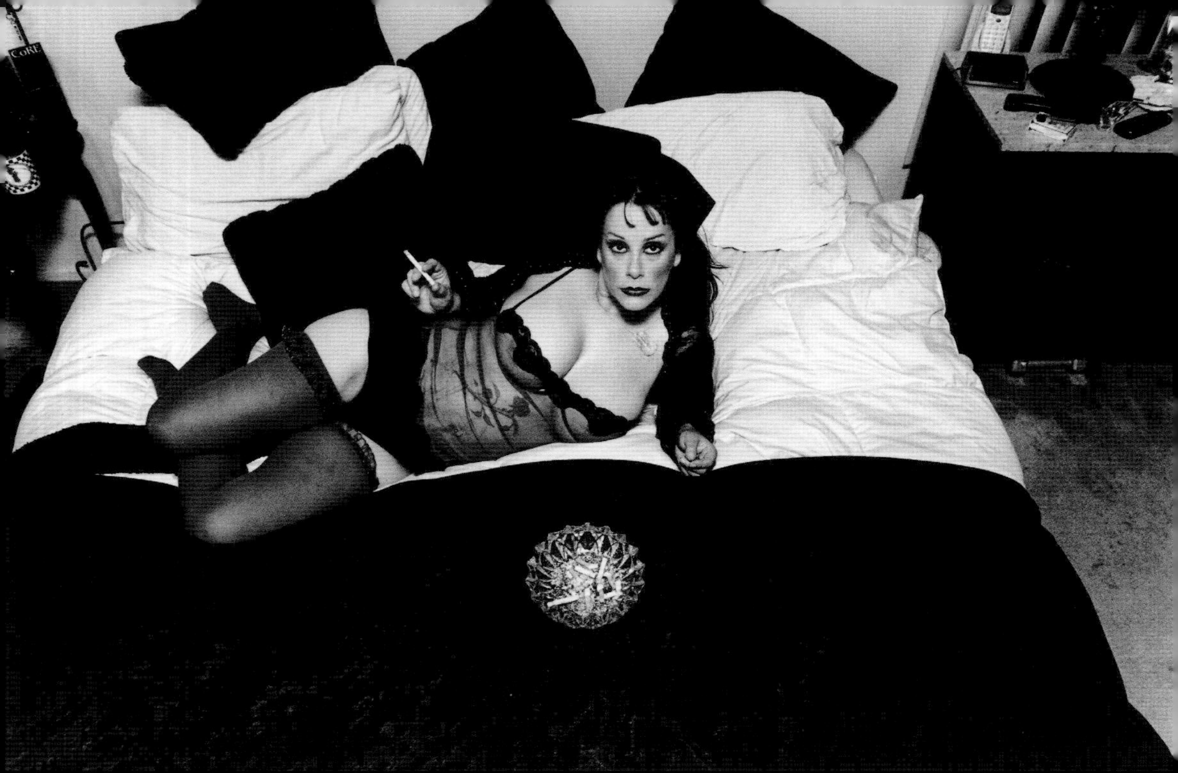

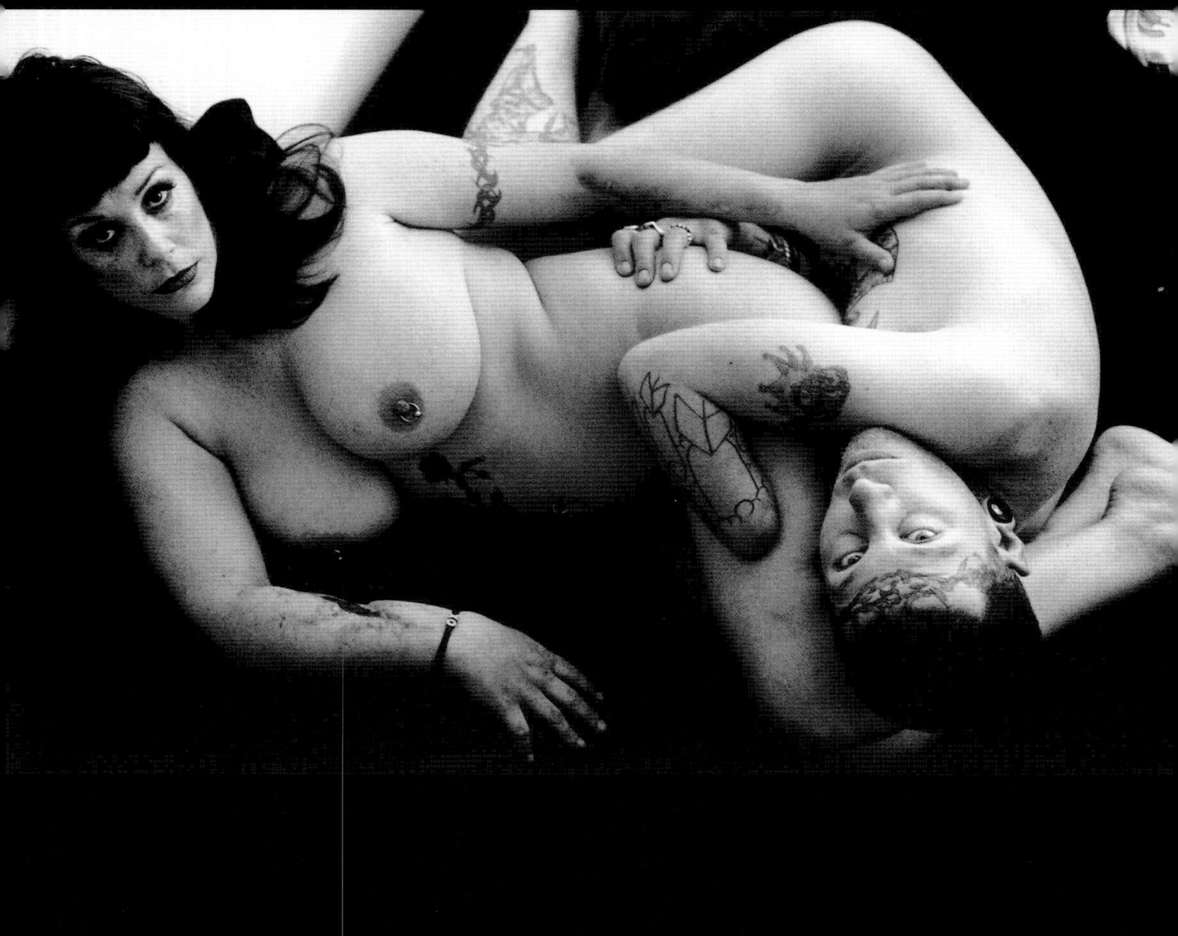

Mistress Sin . Mistress Sin & Nub

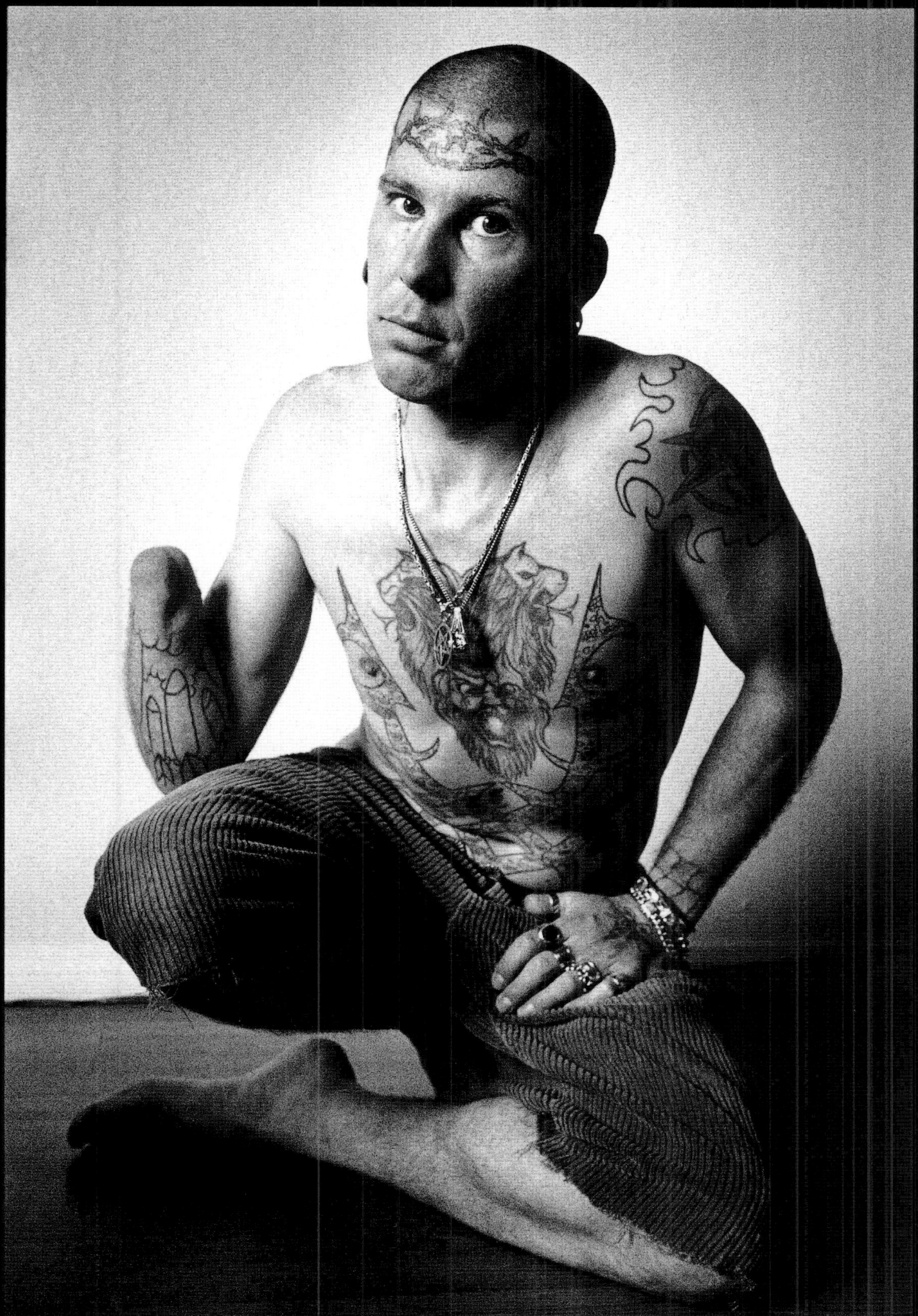

Nub

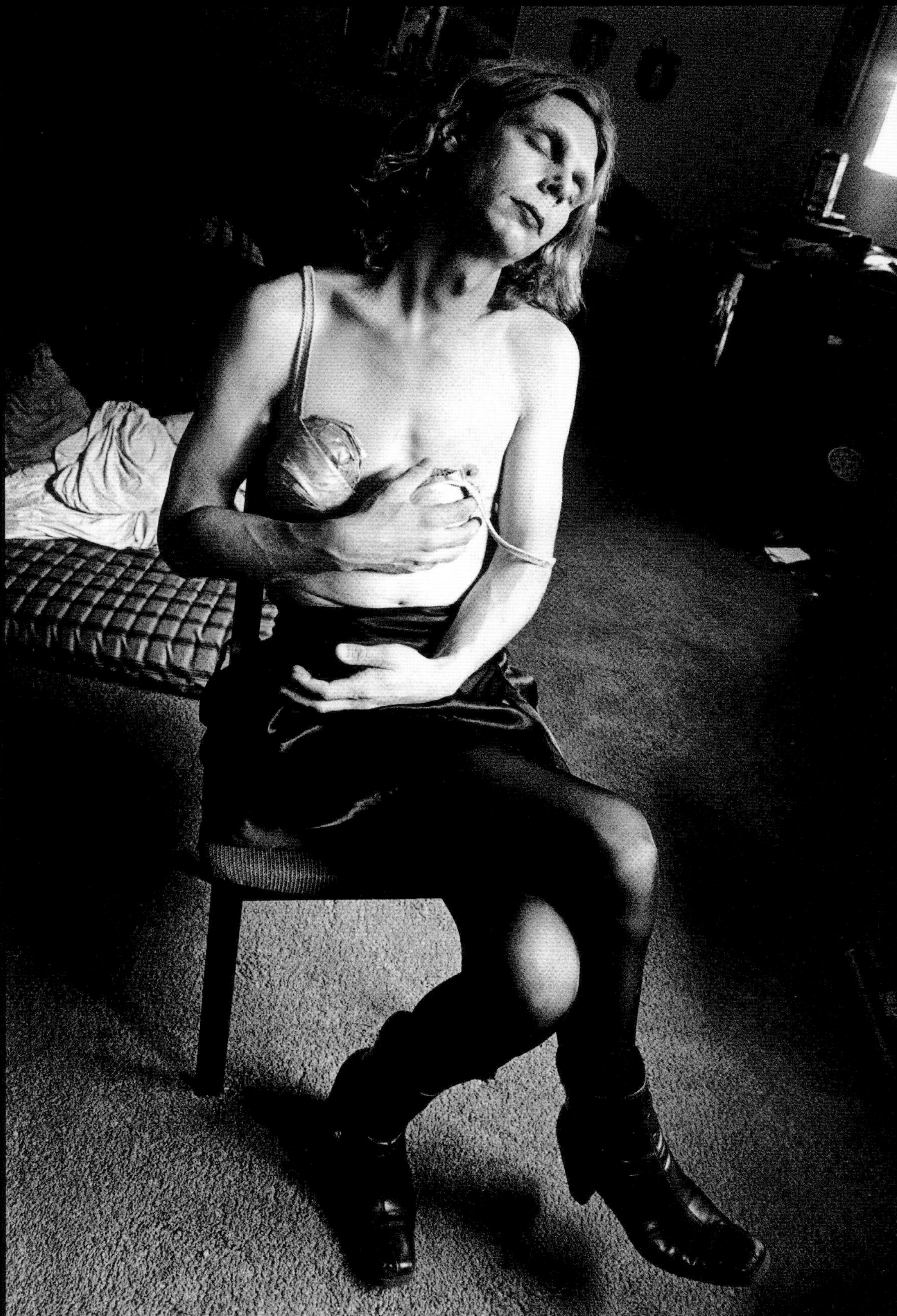

Sissy Girl Shaky

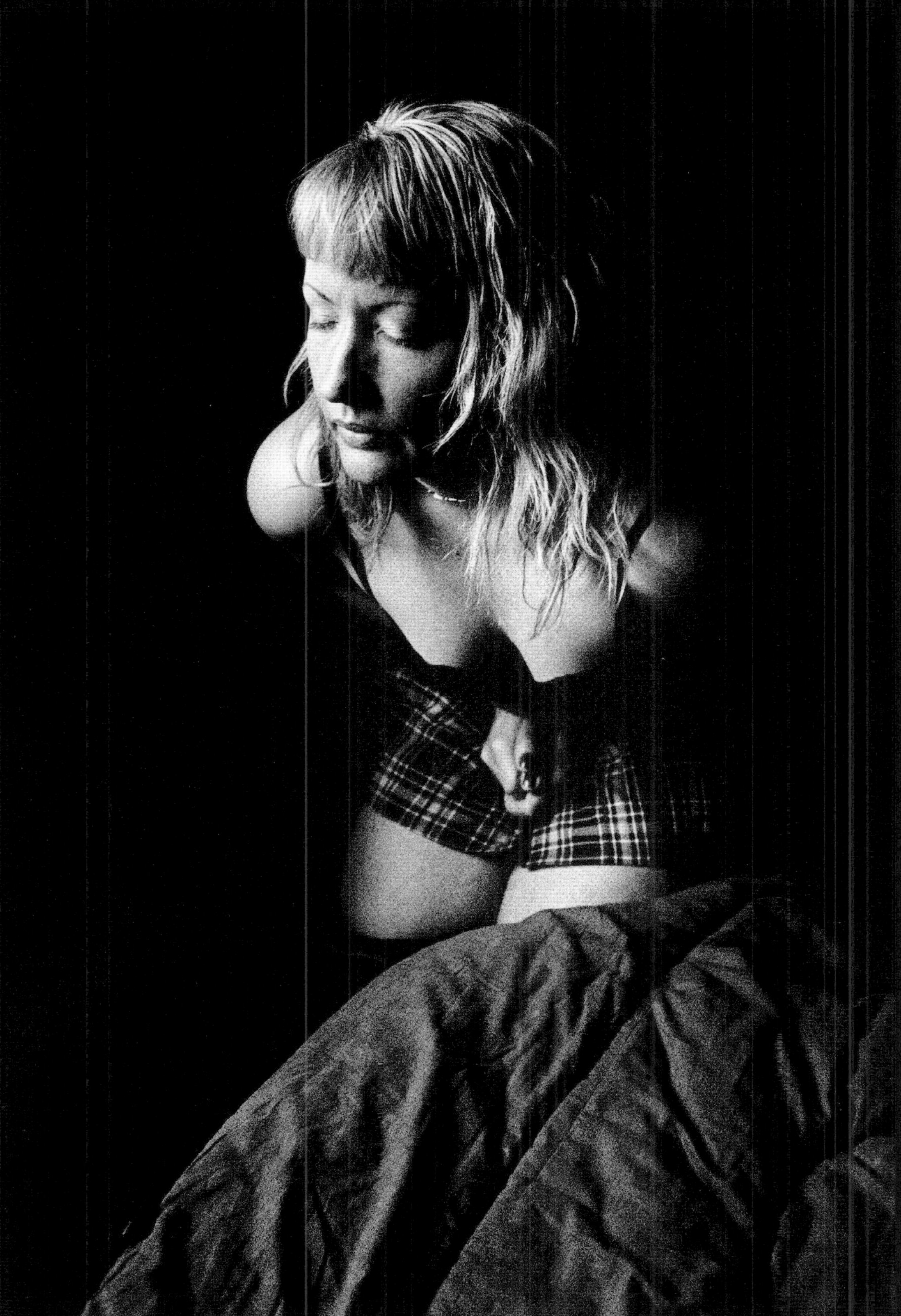

Dawn

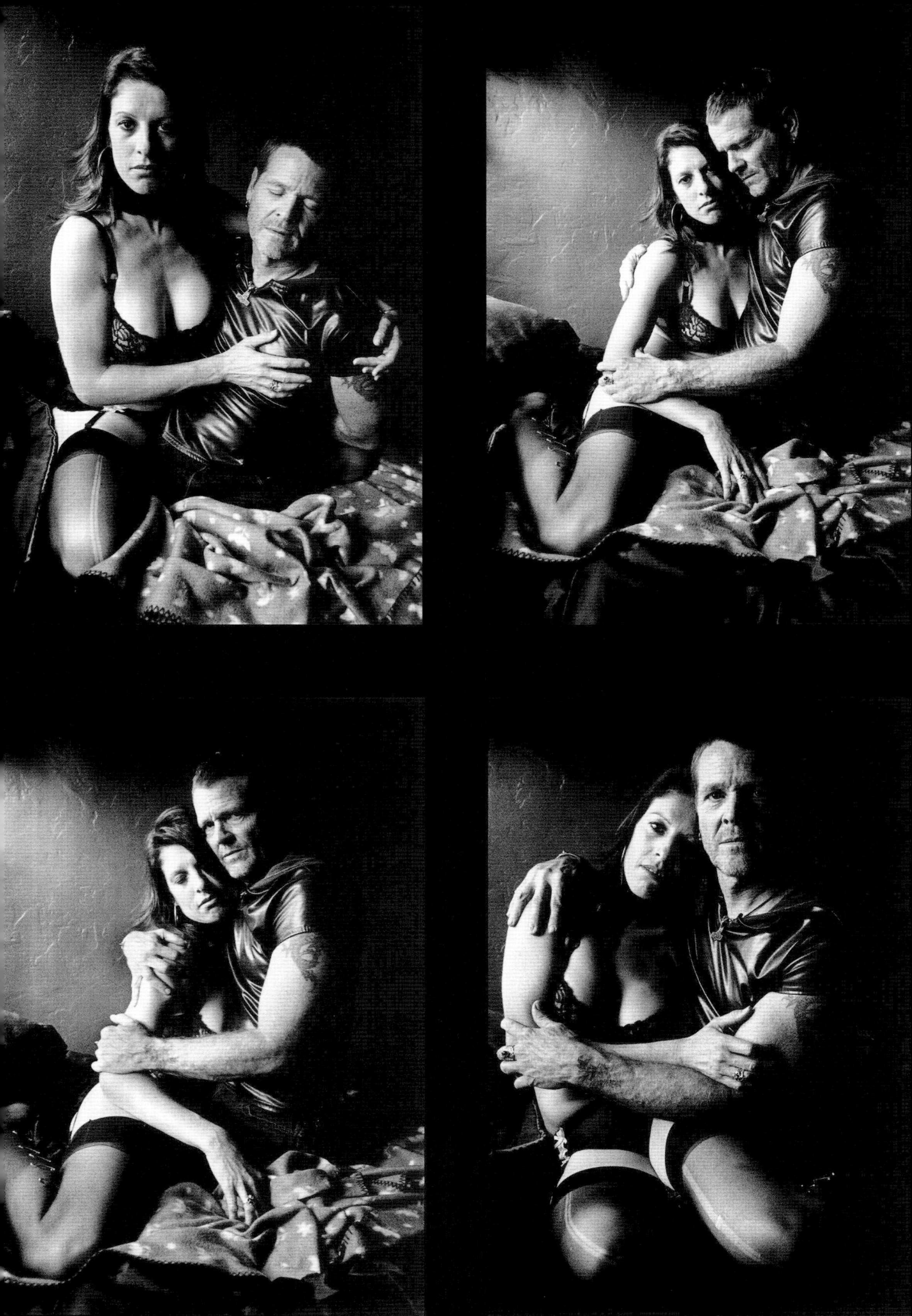

Bill & Marie

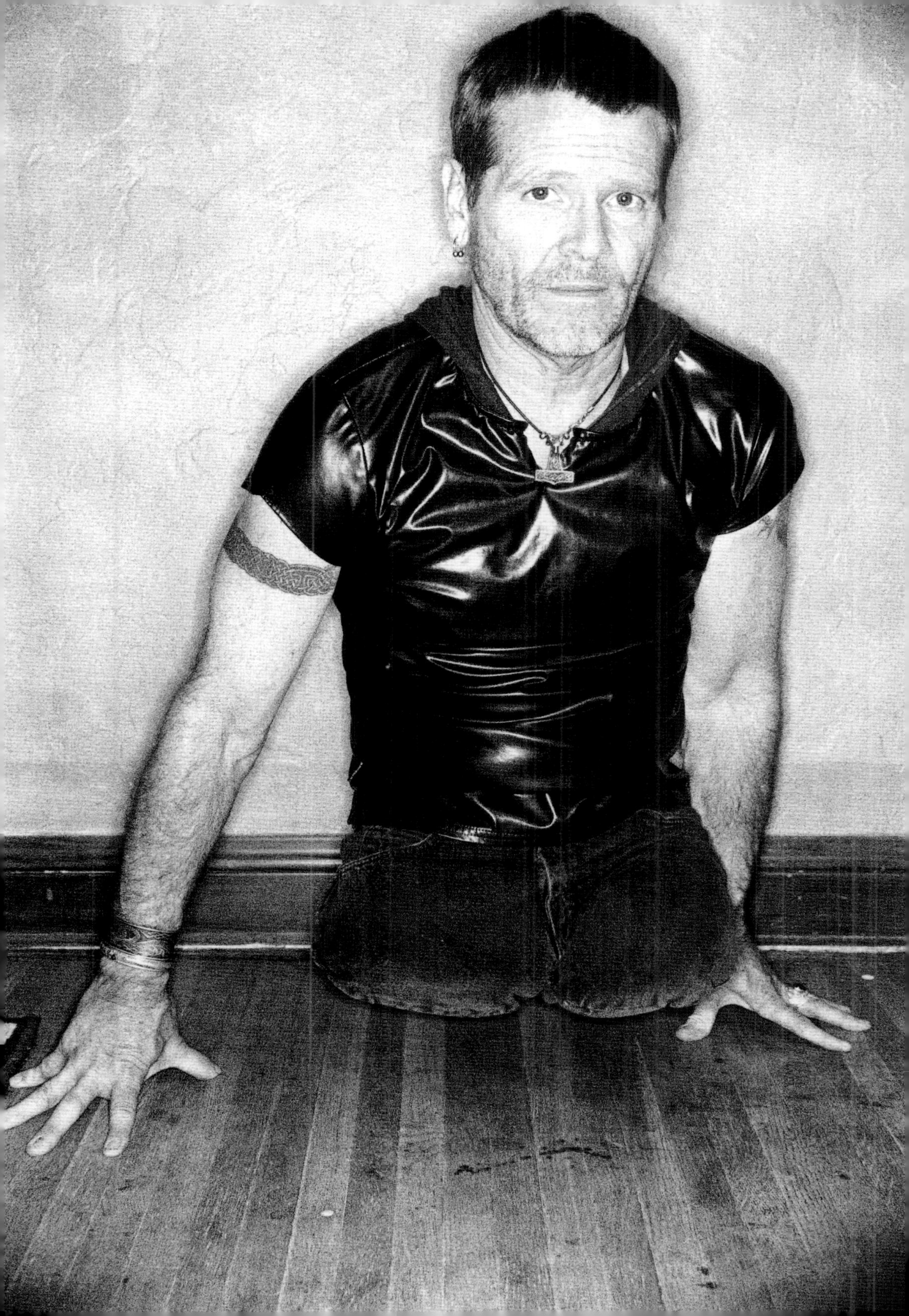

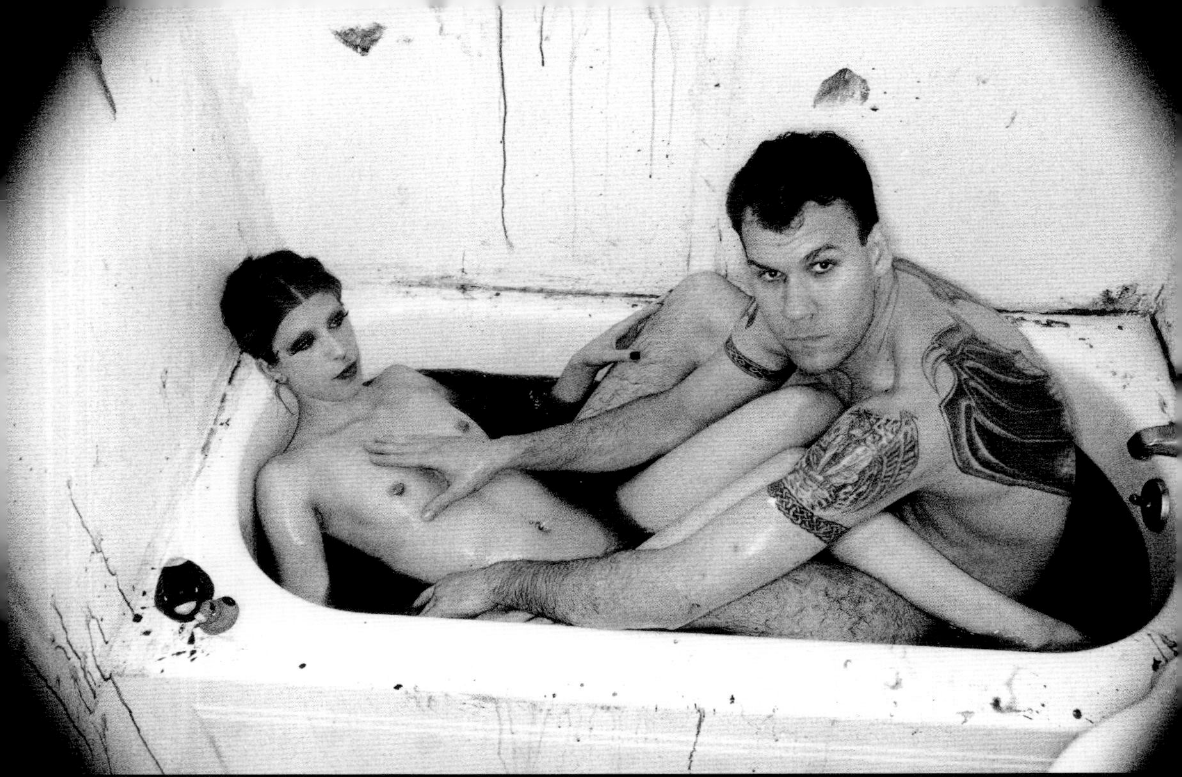

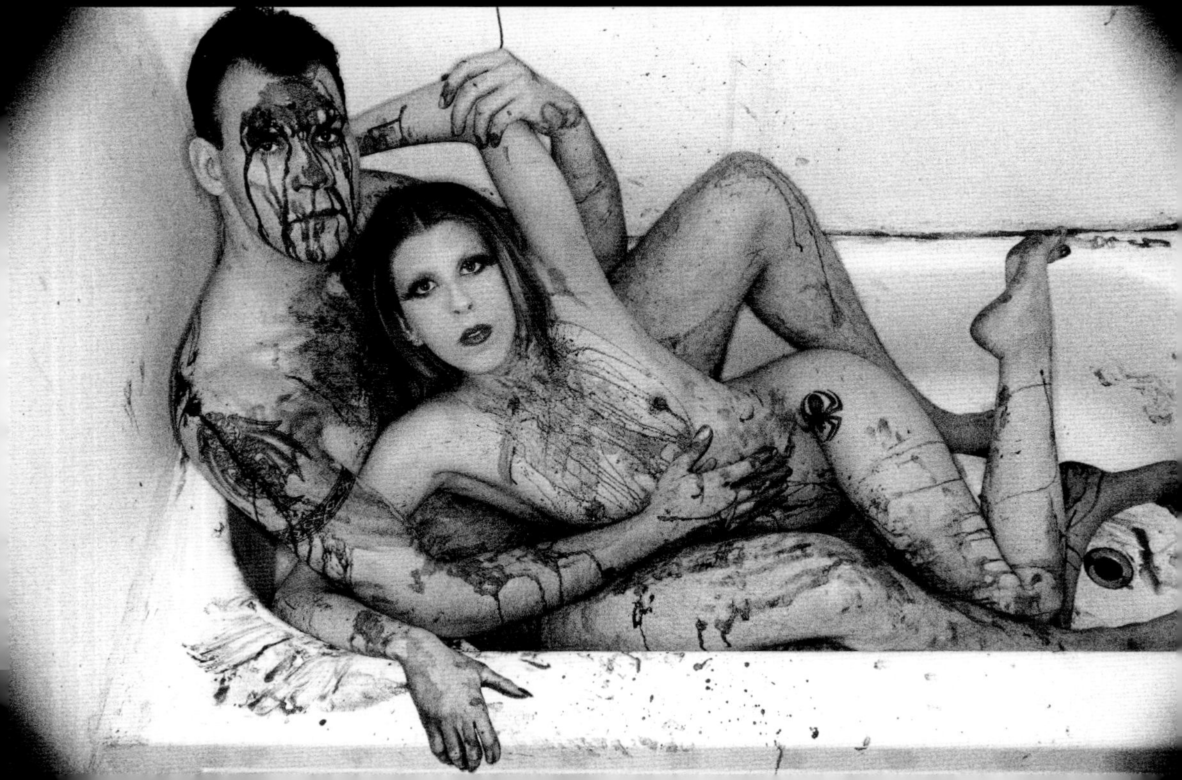

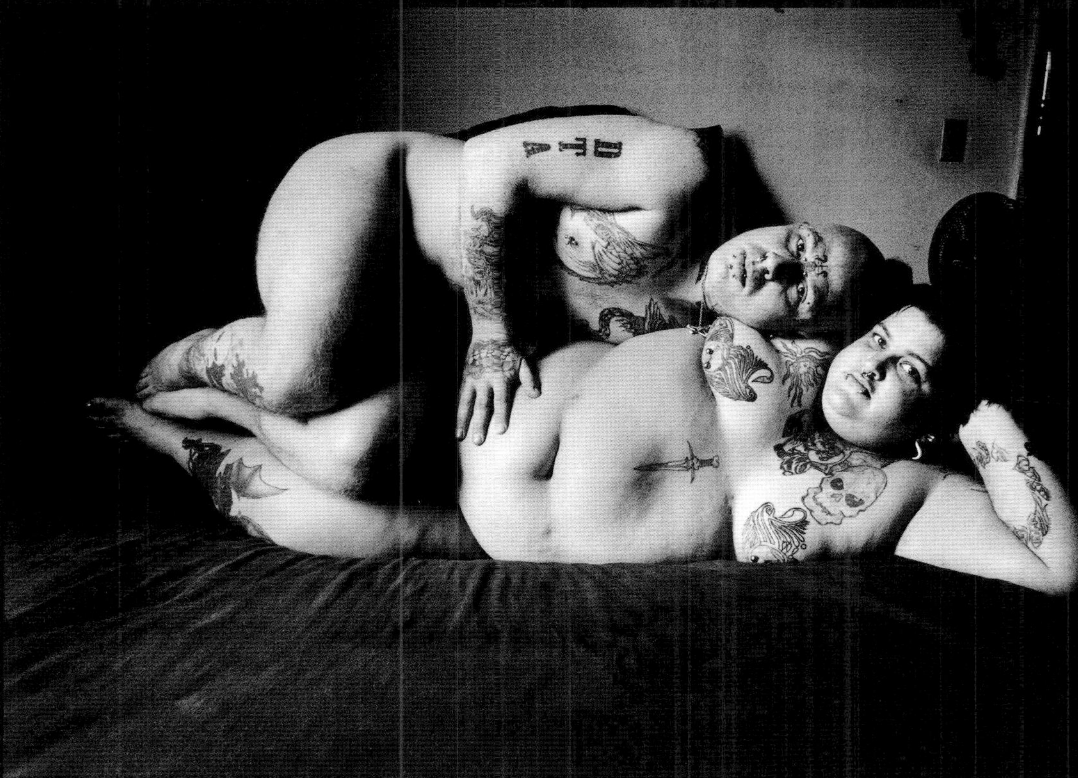

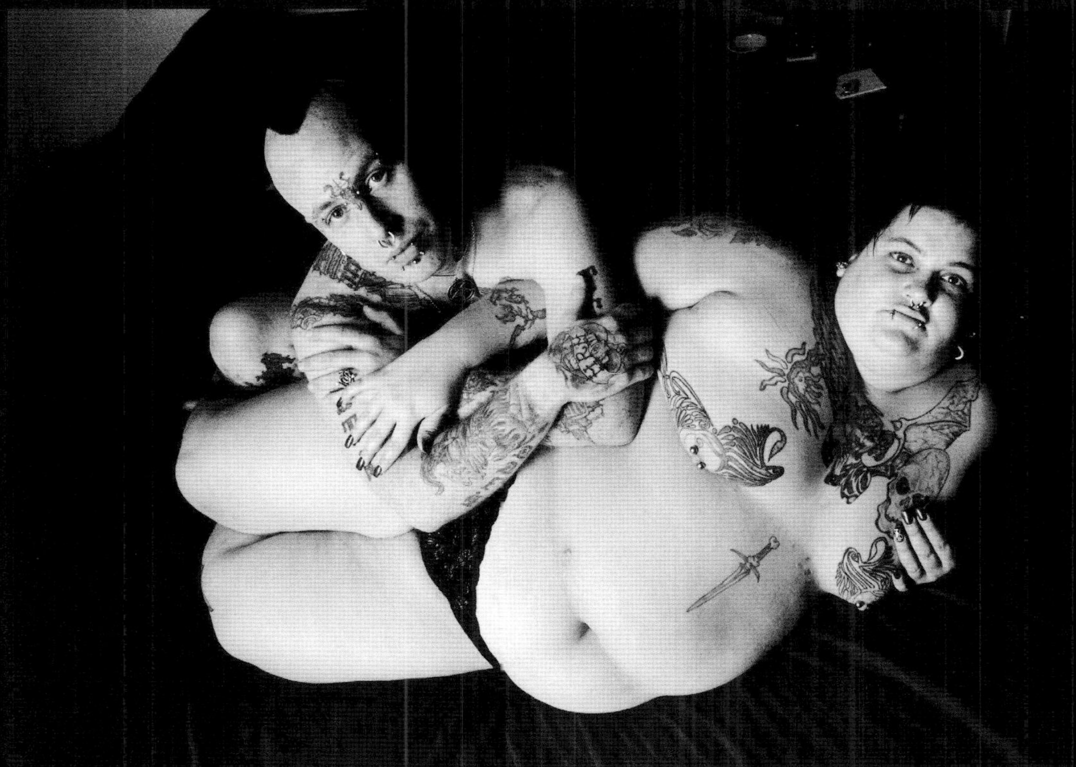

Sonny & Amber

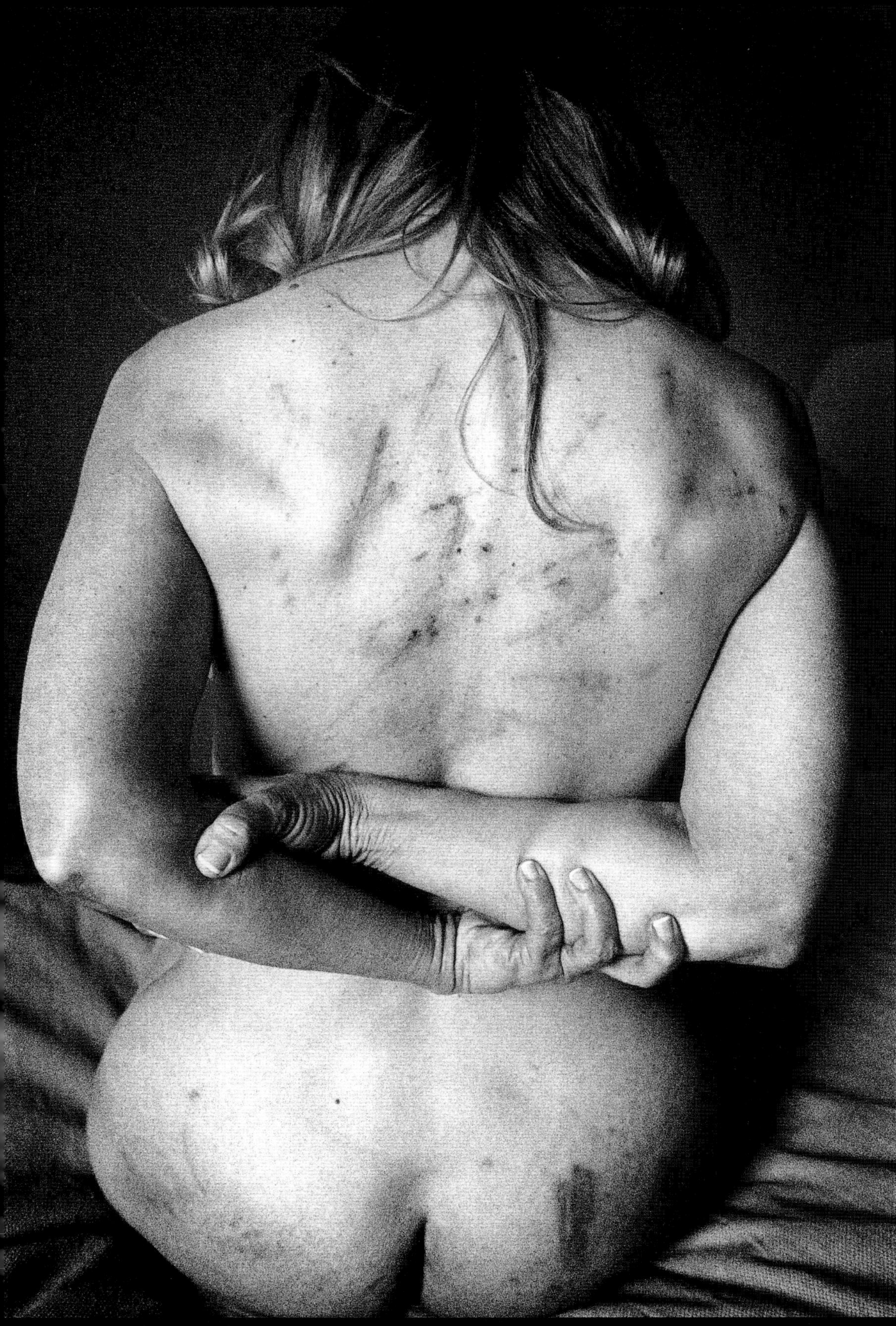

Ann

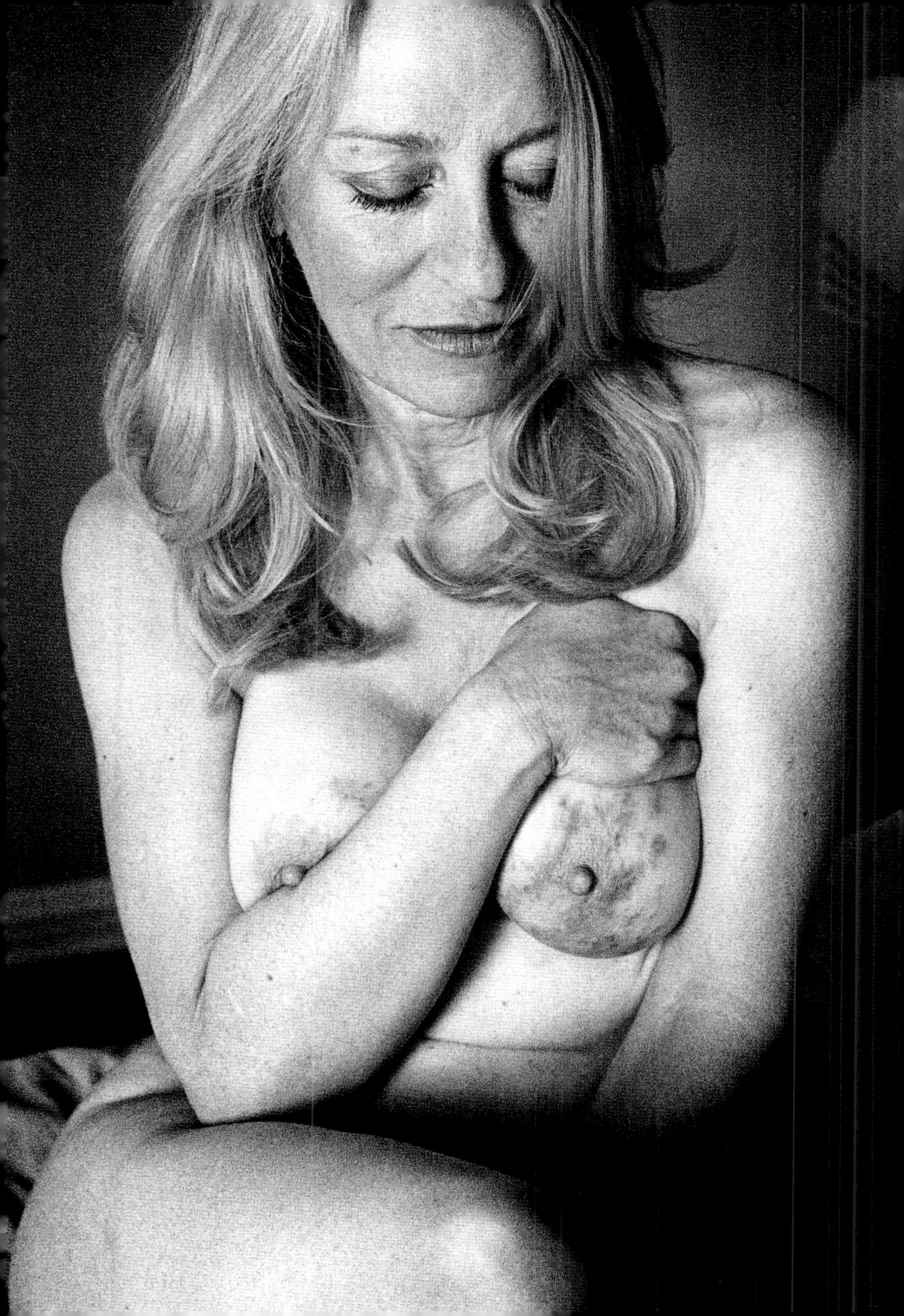

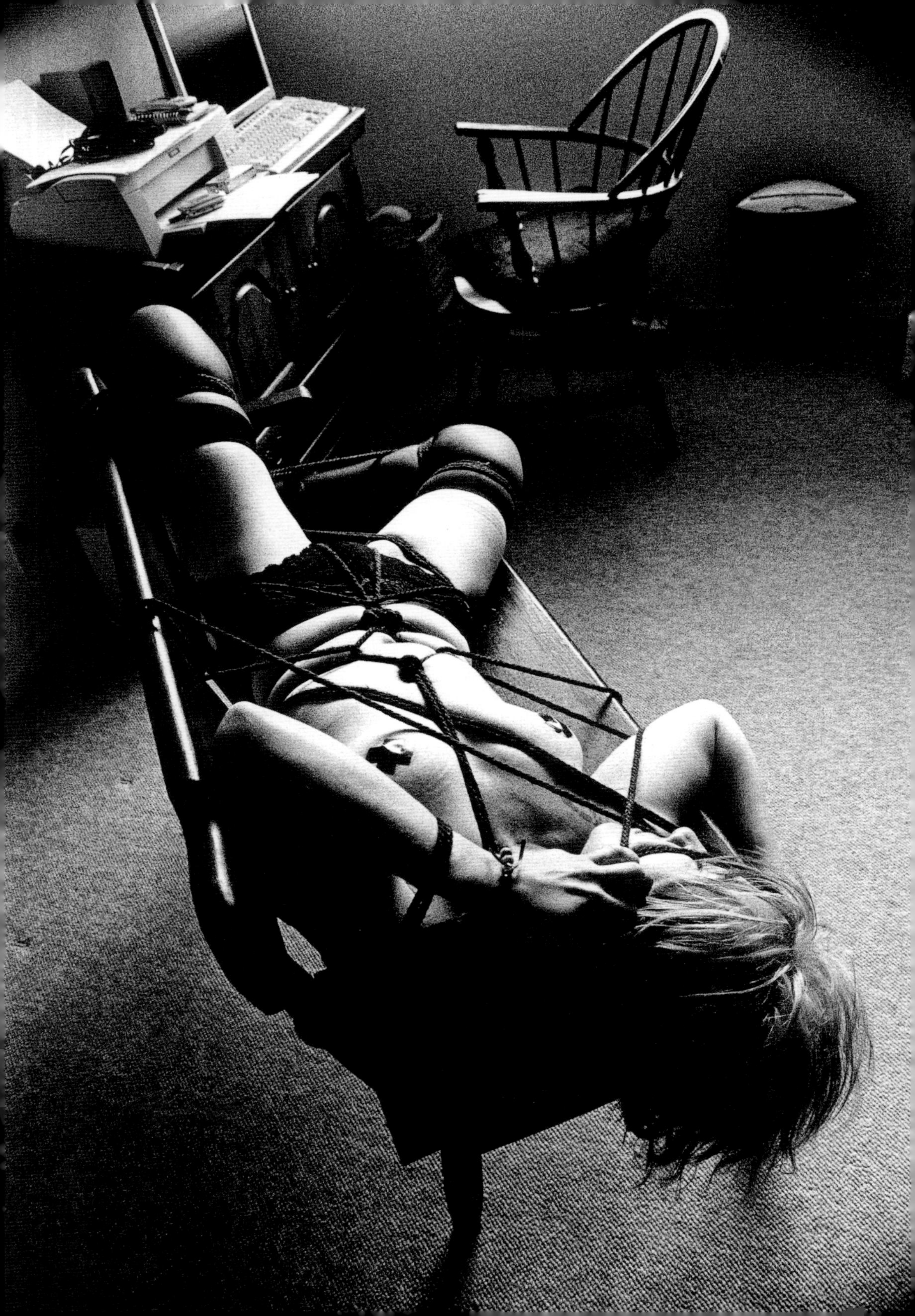

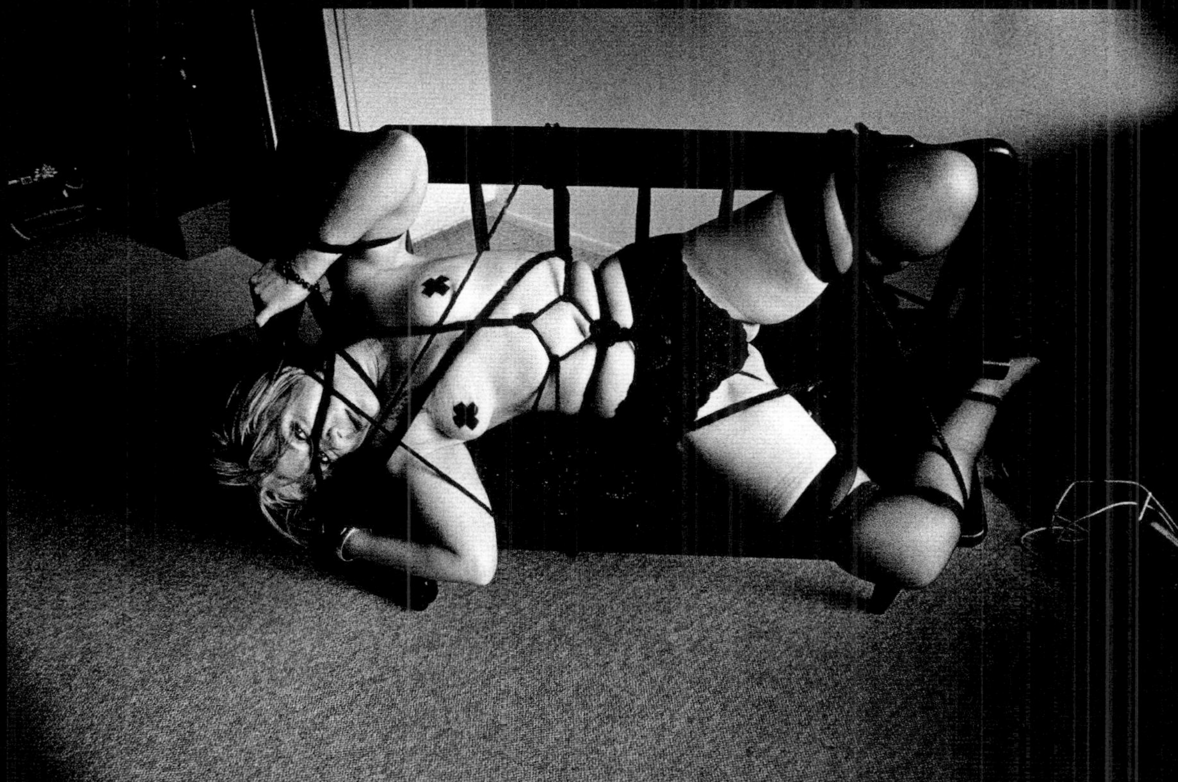

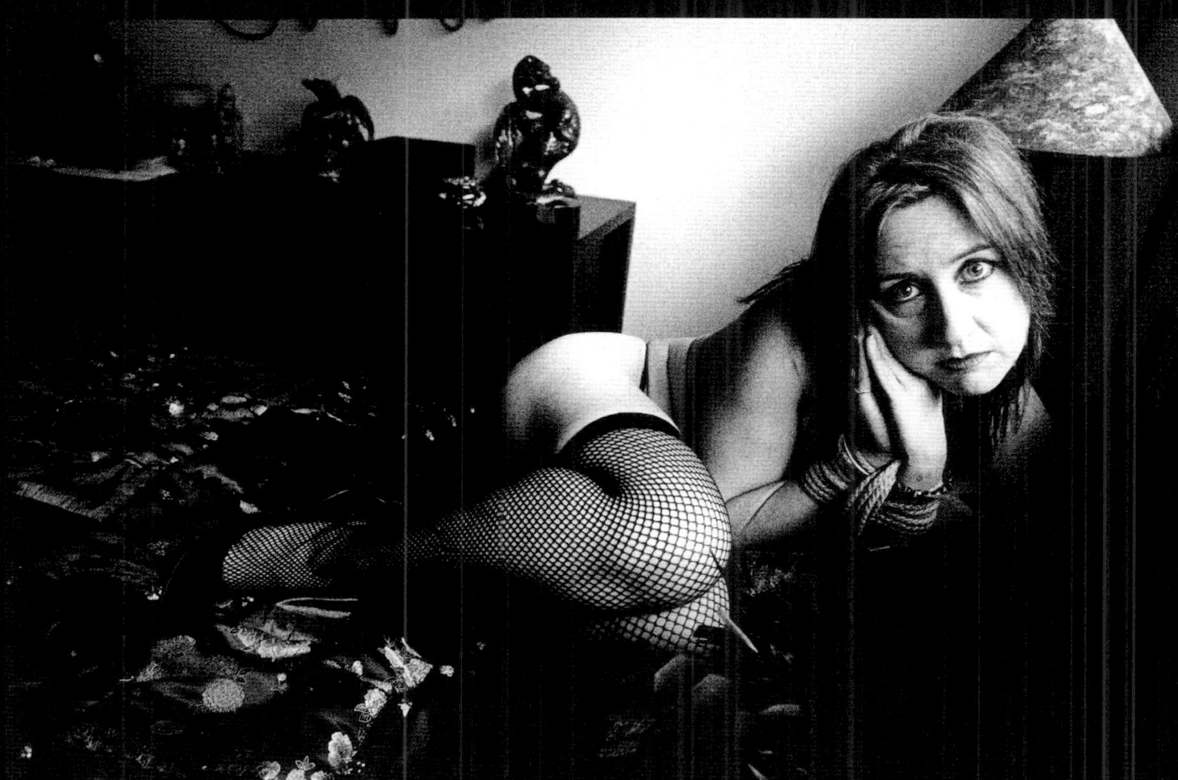

Alchemy

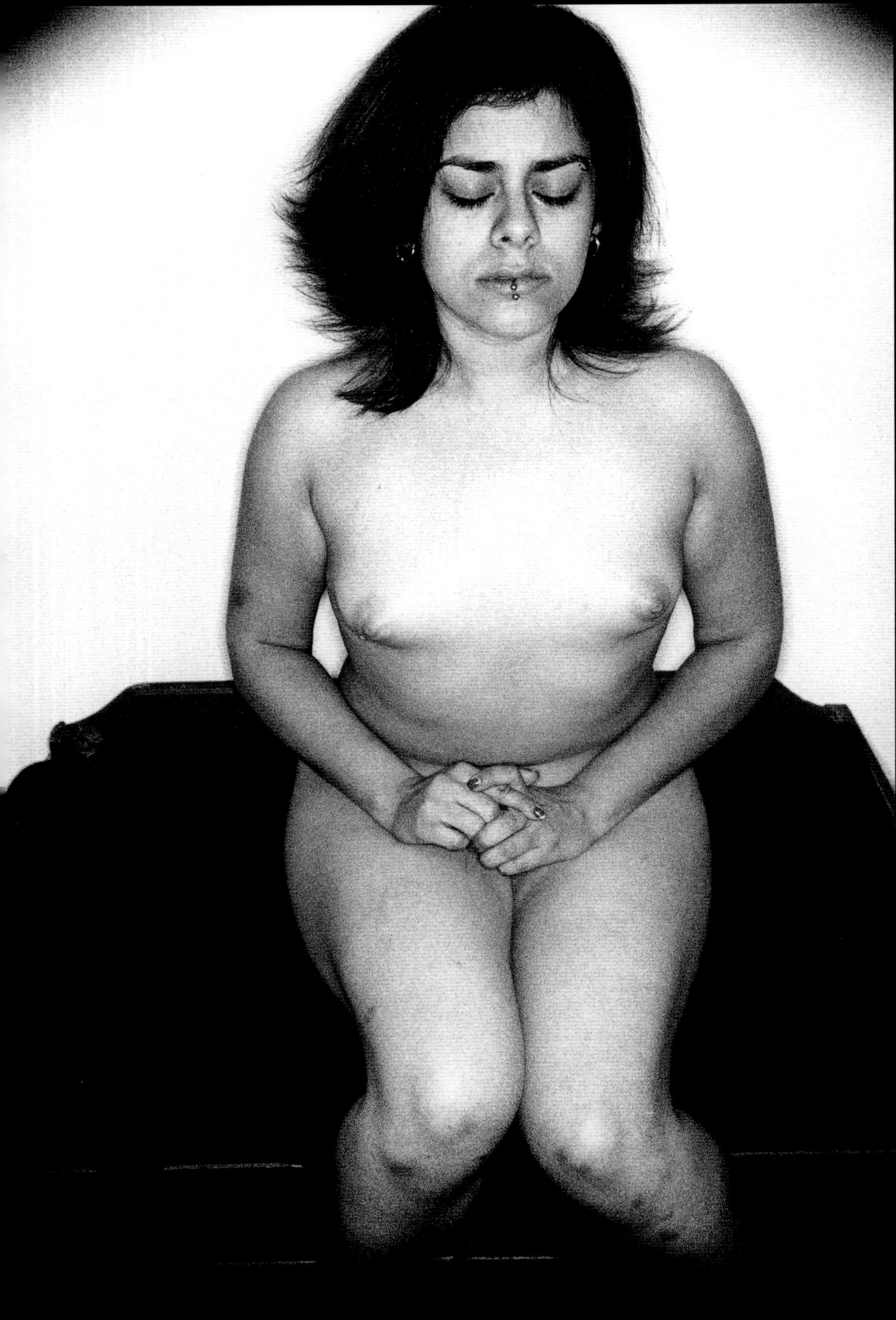

April

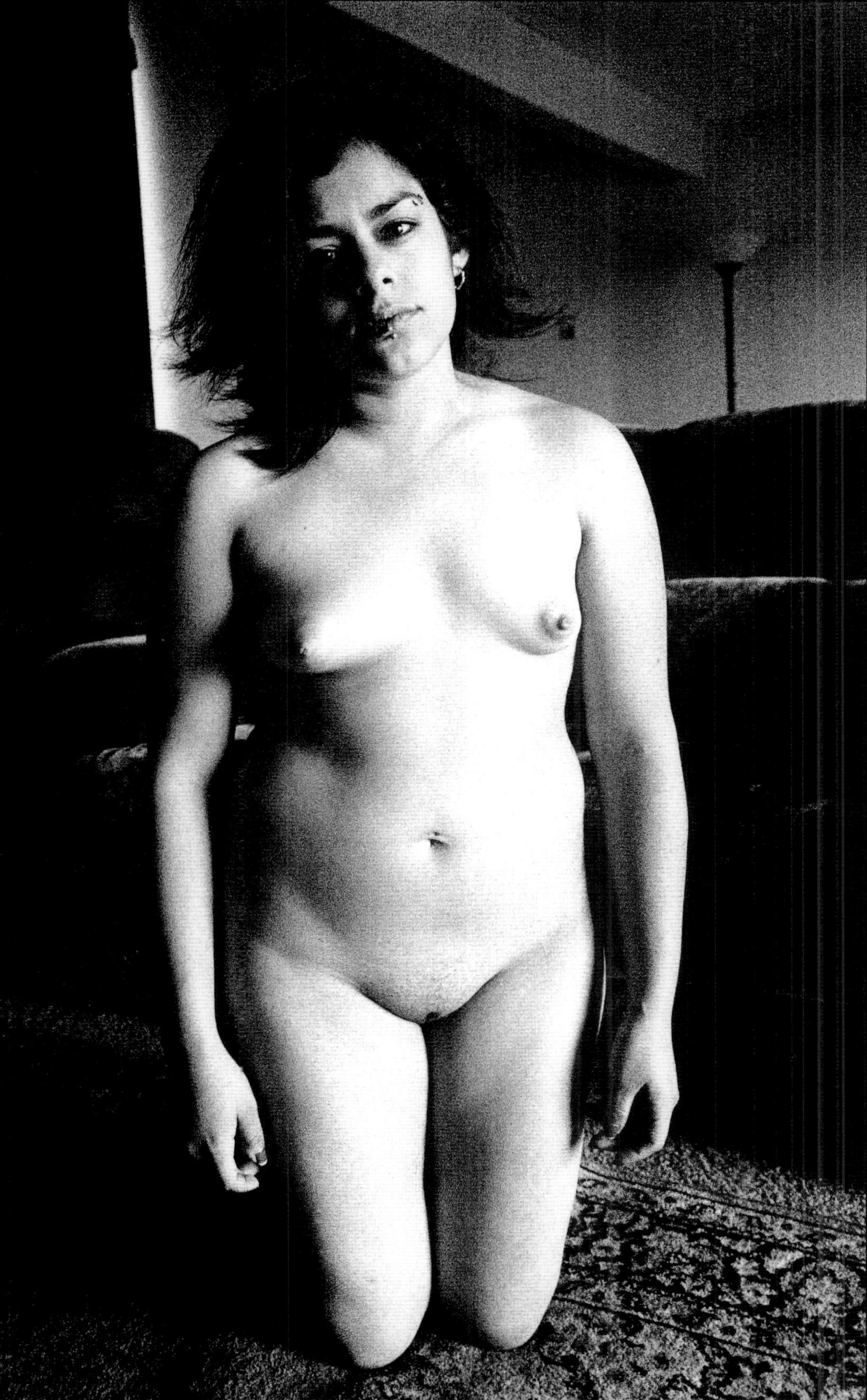

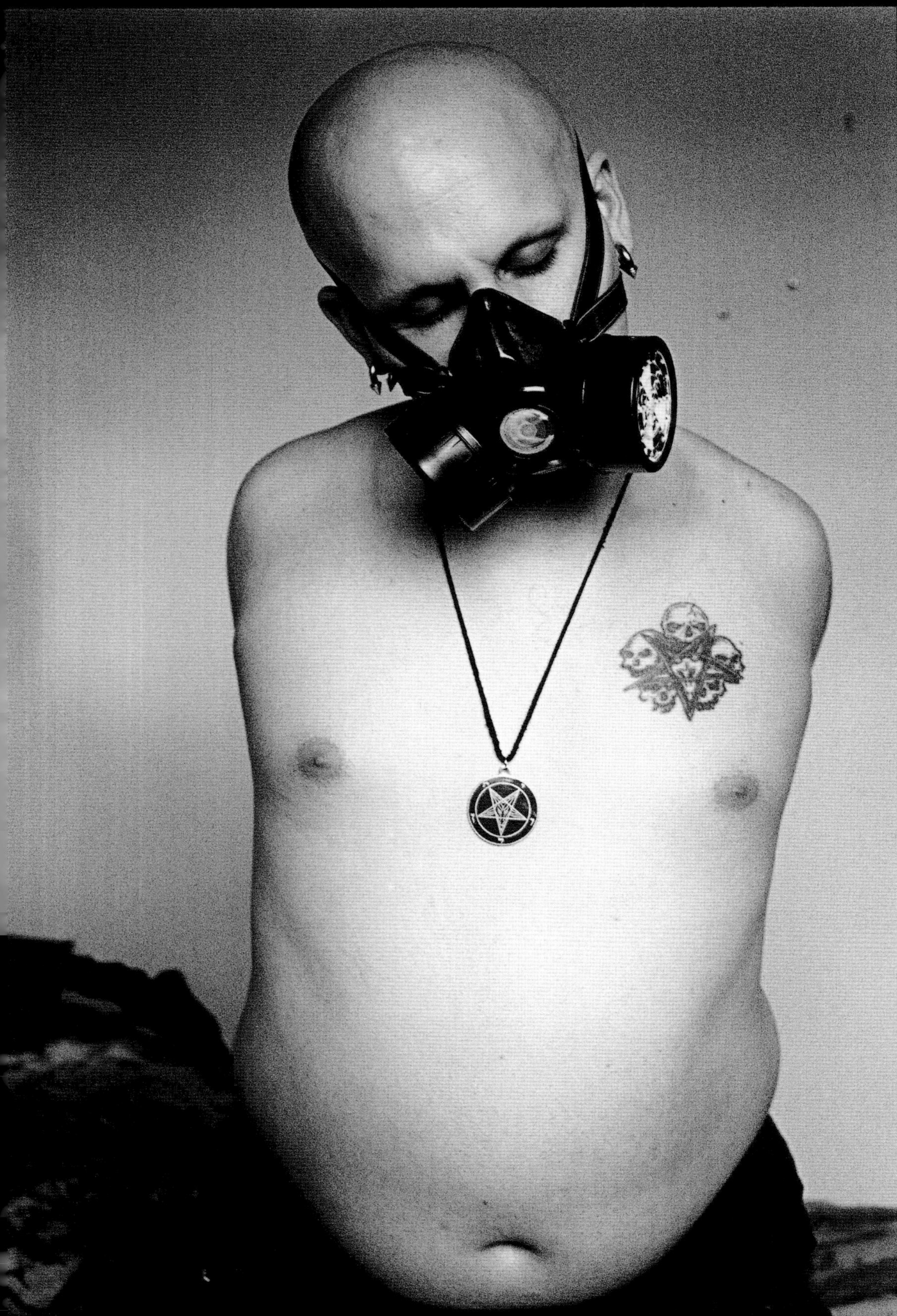

Boon

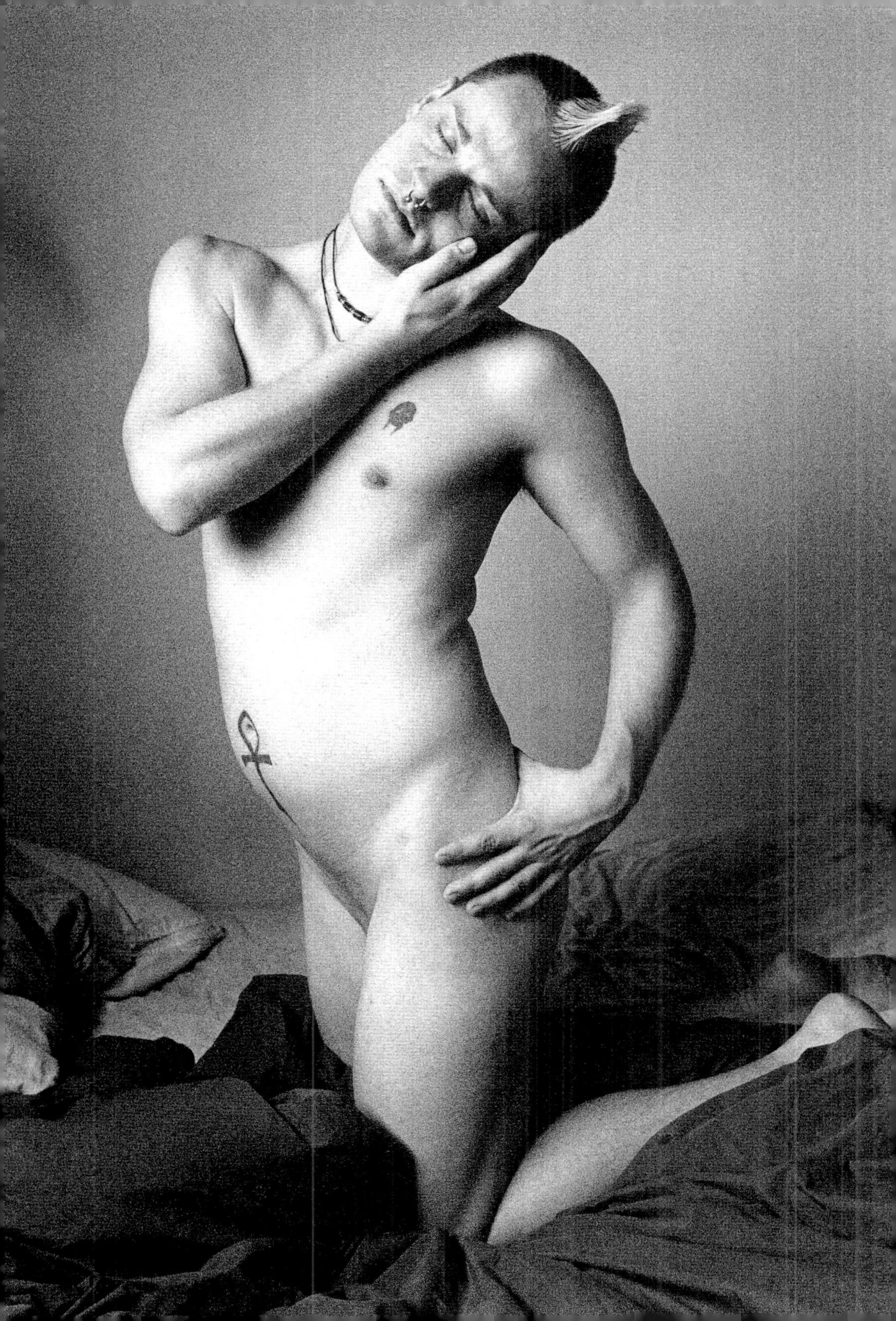

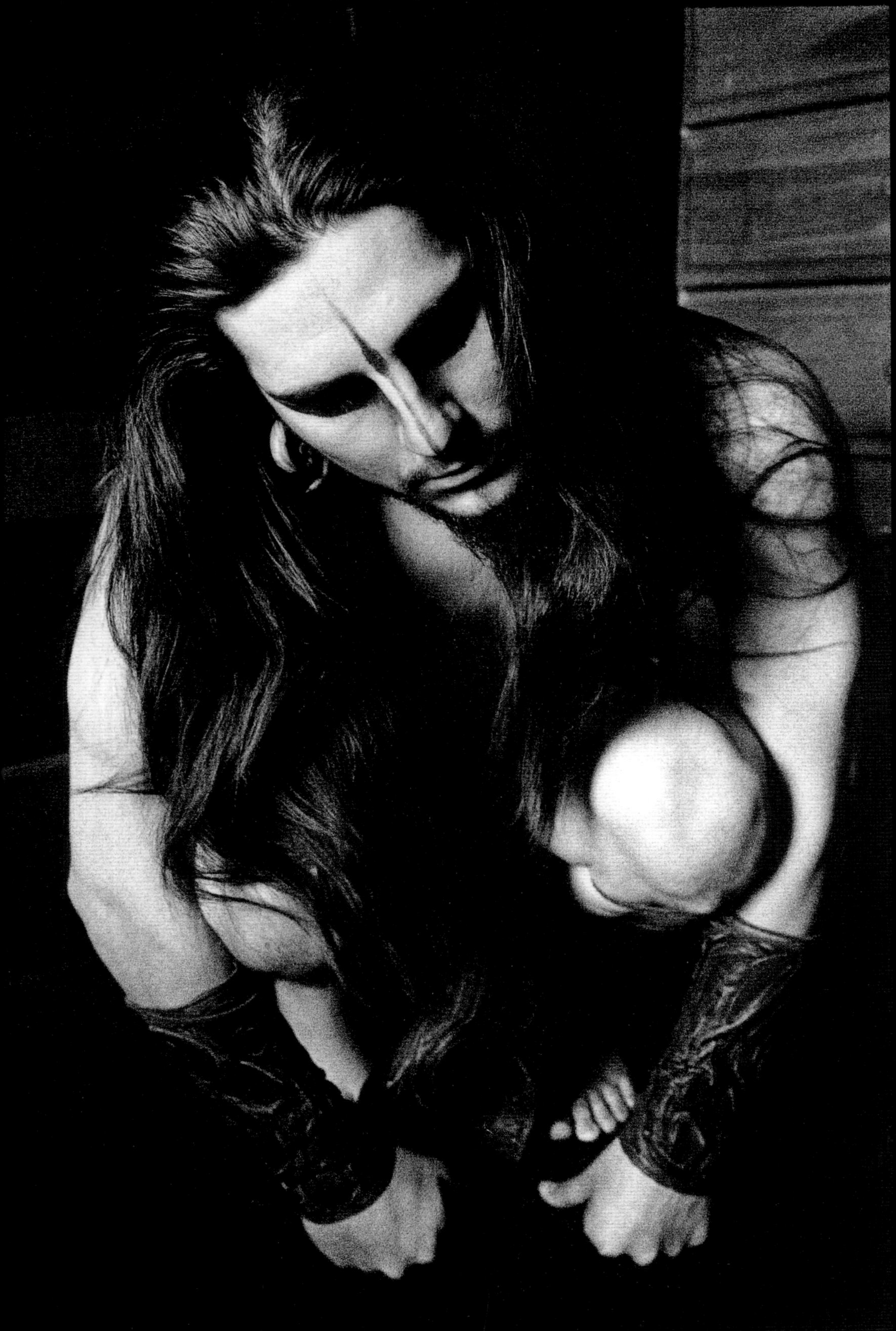

Cosmo

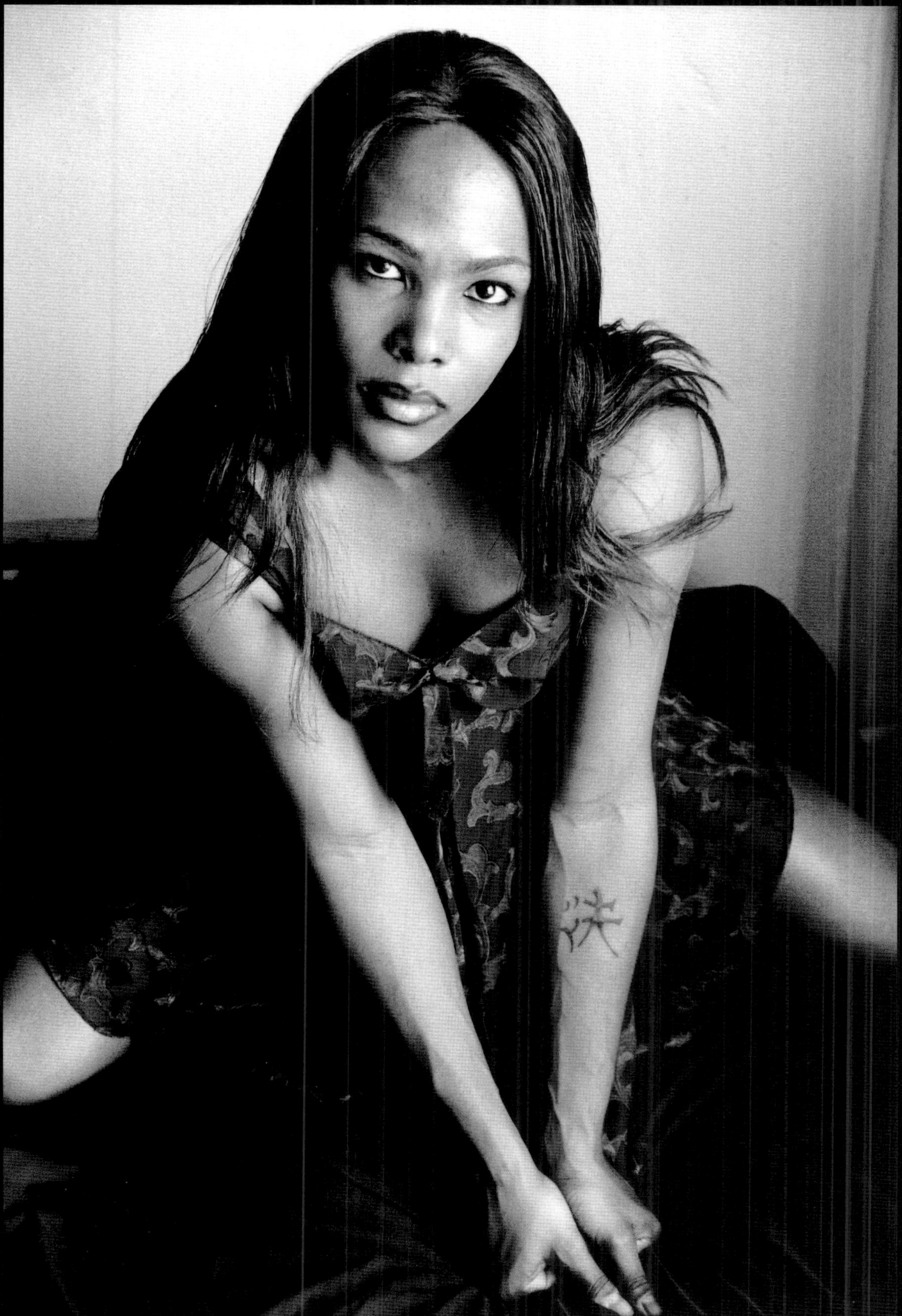

Nahshon

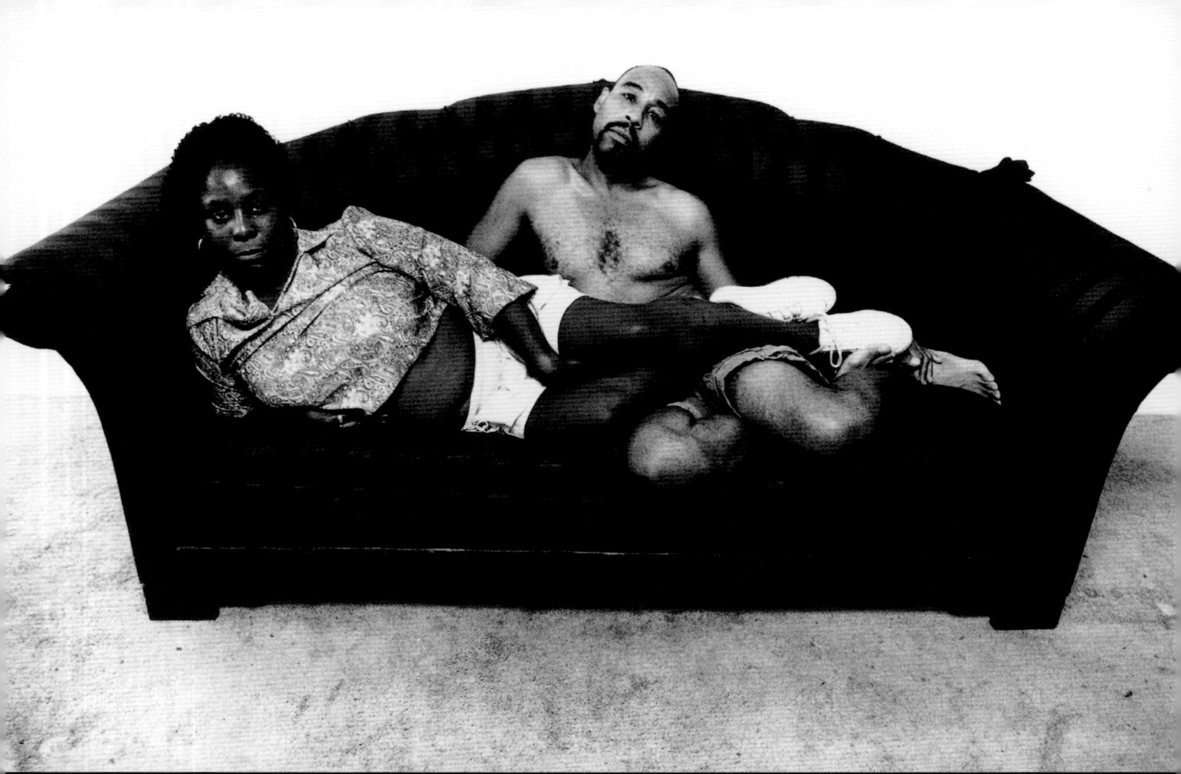

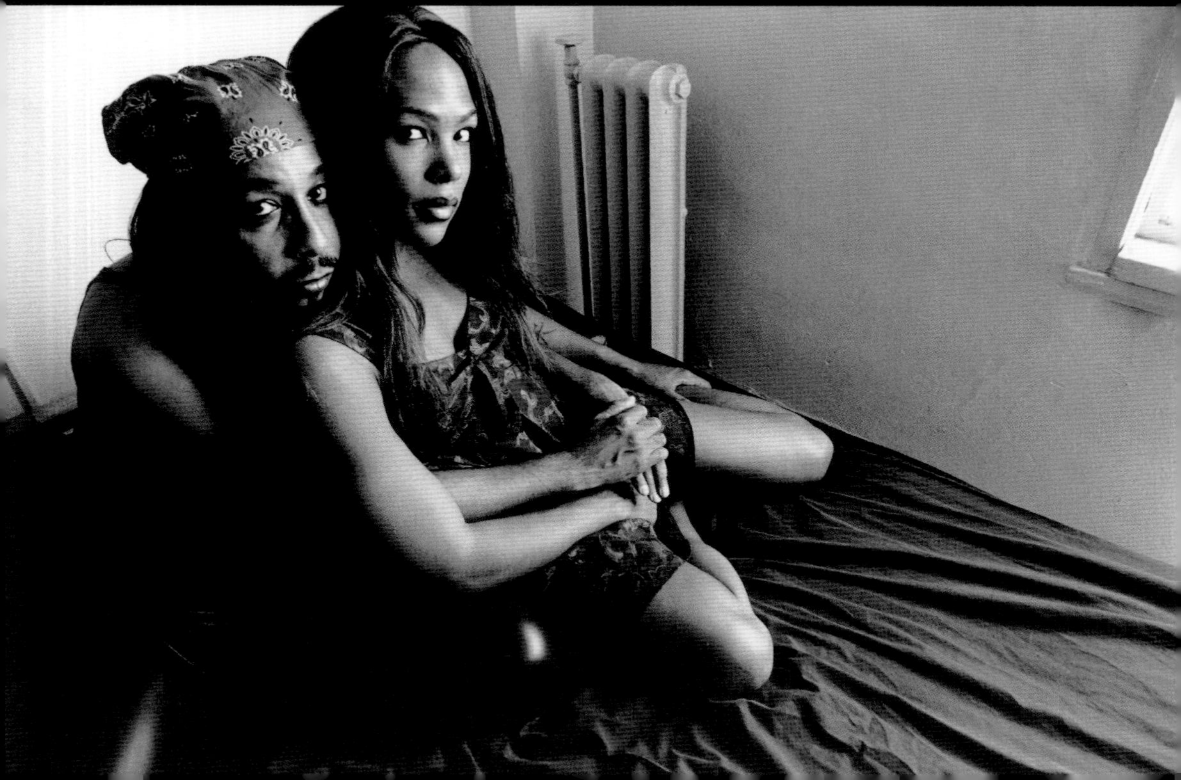

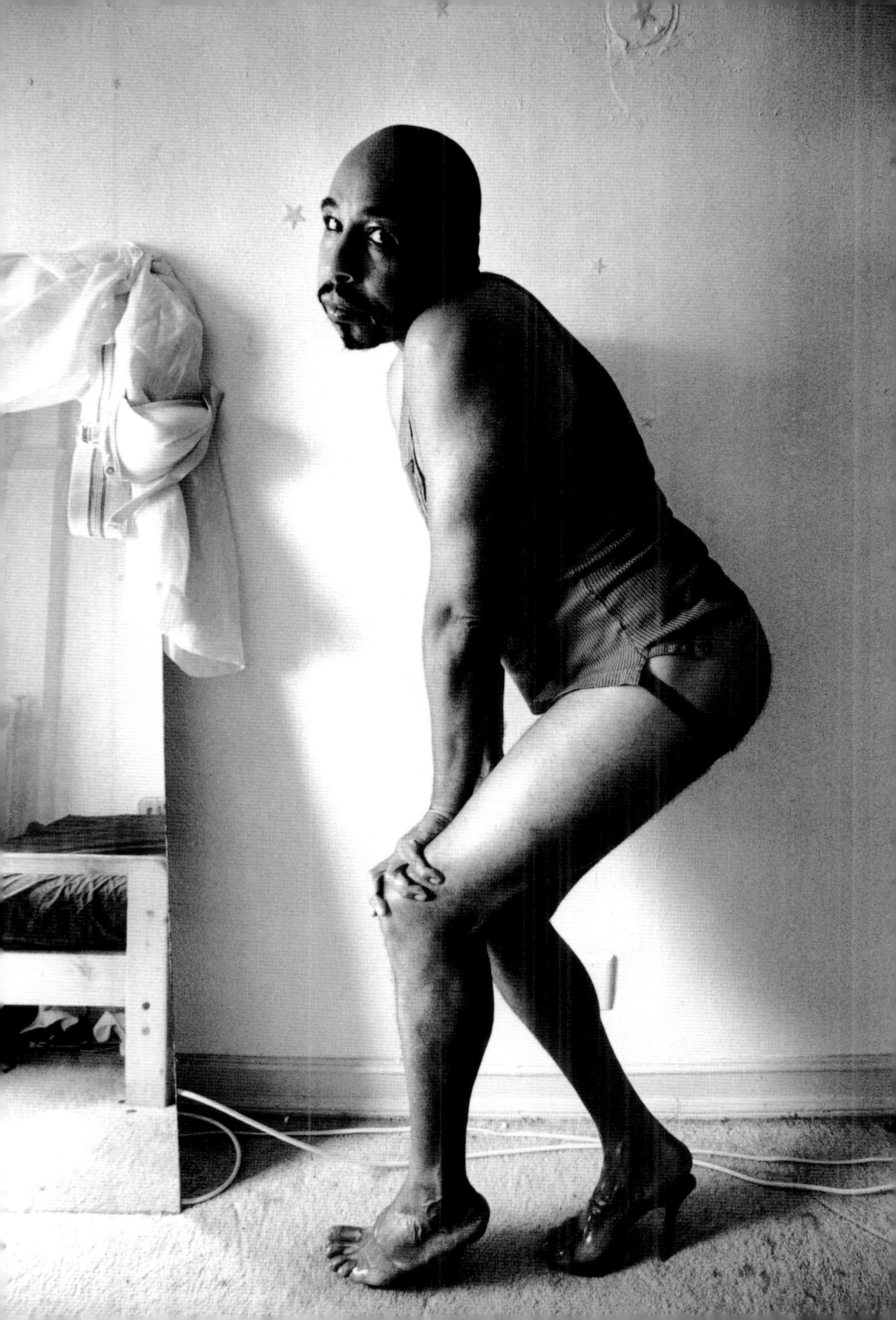

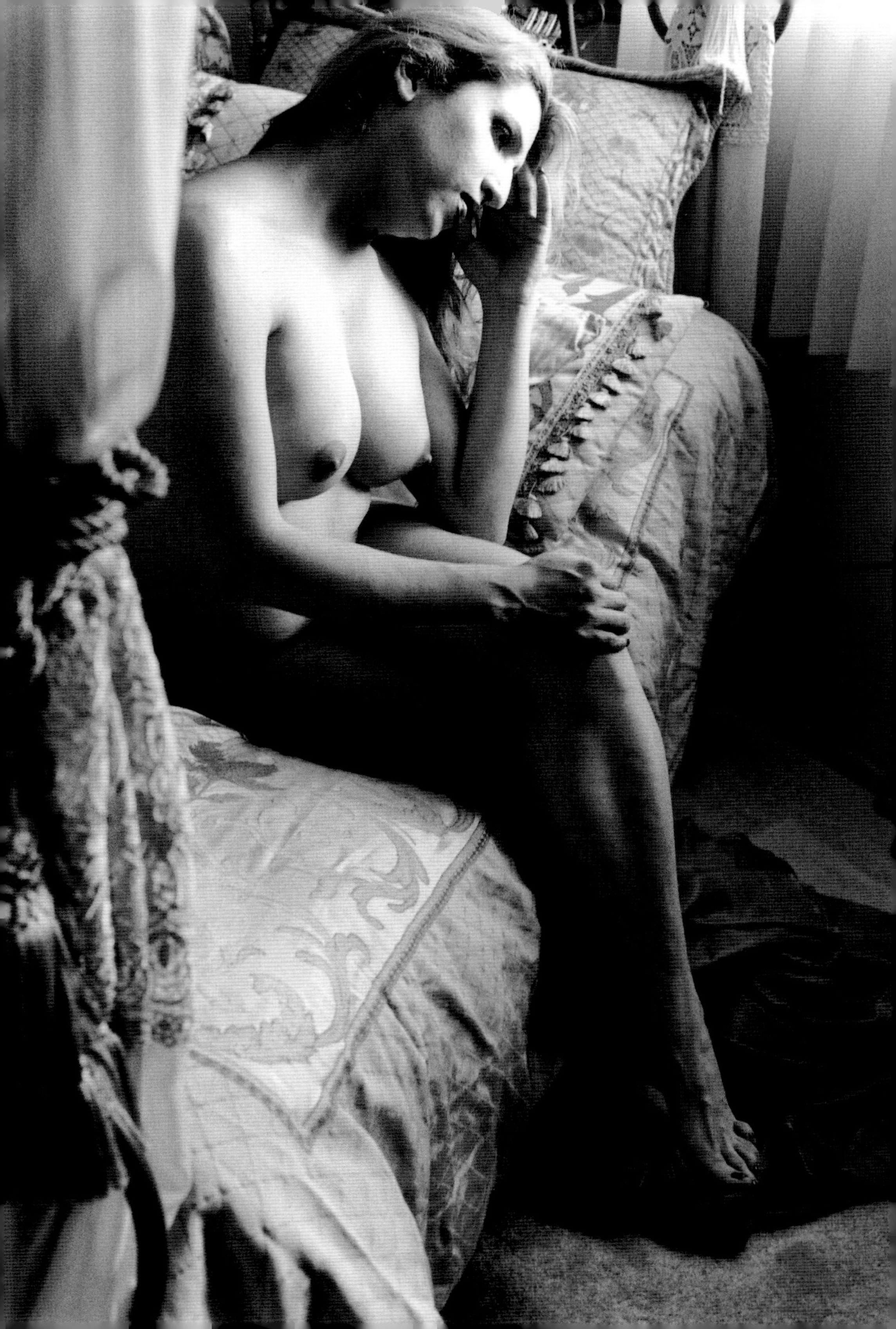

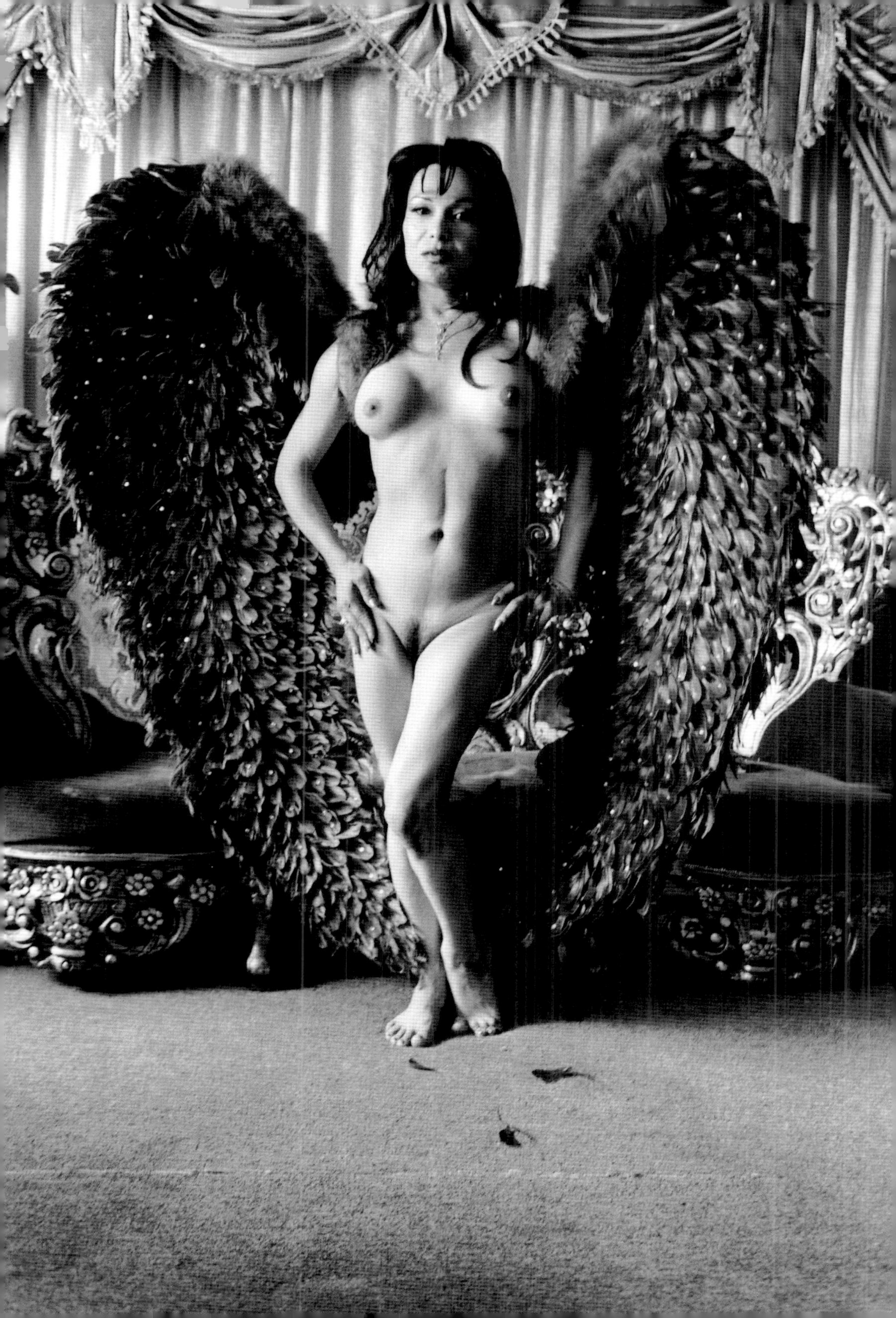

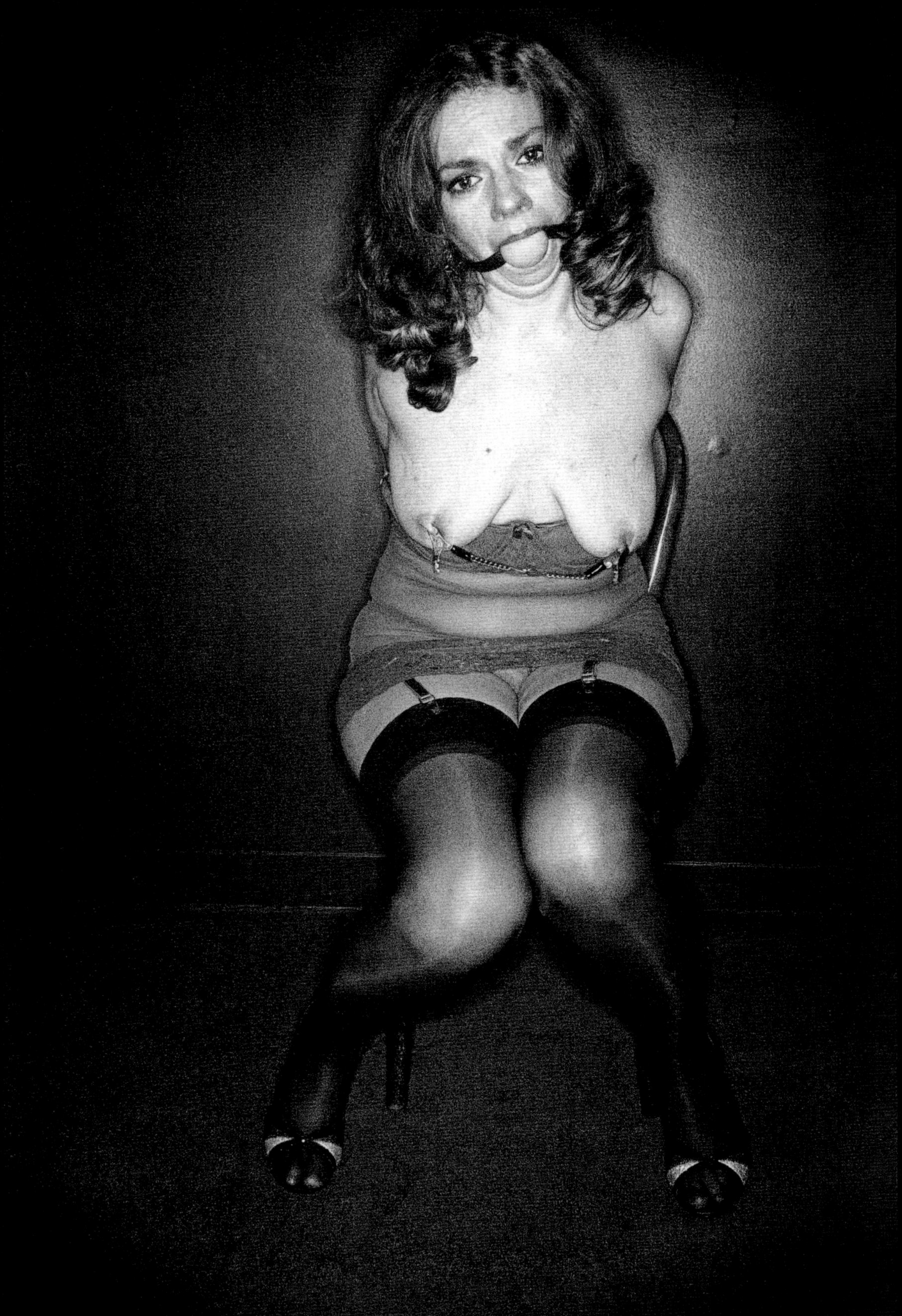

Inna

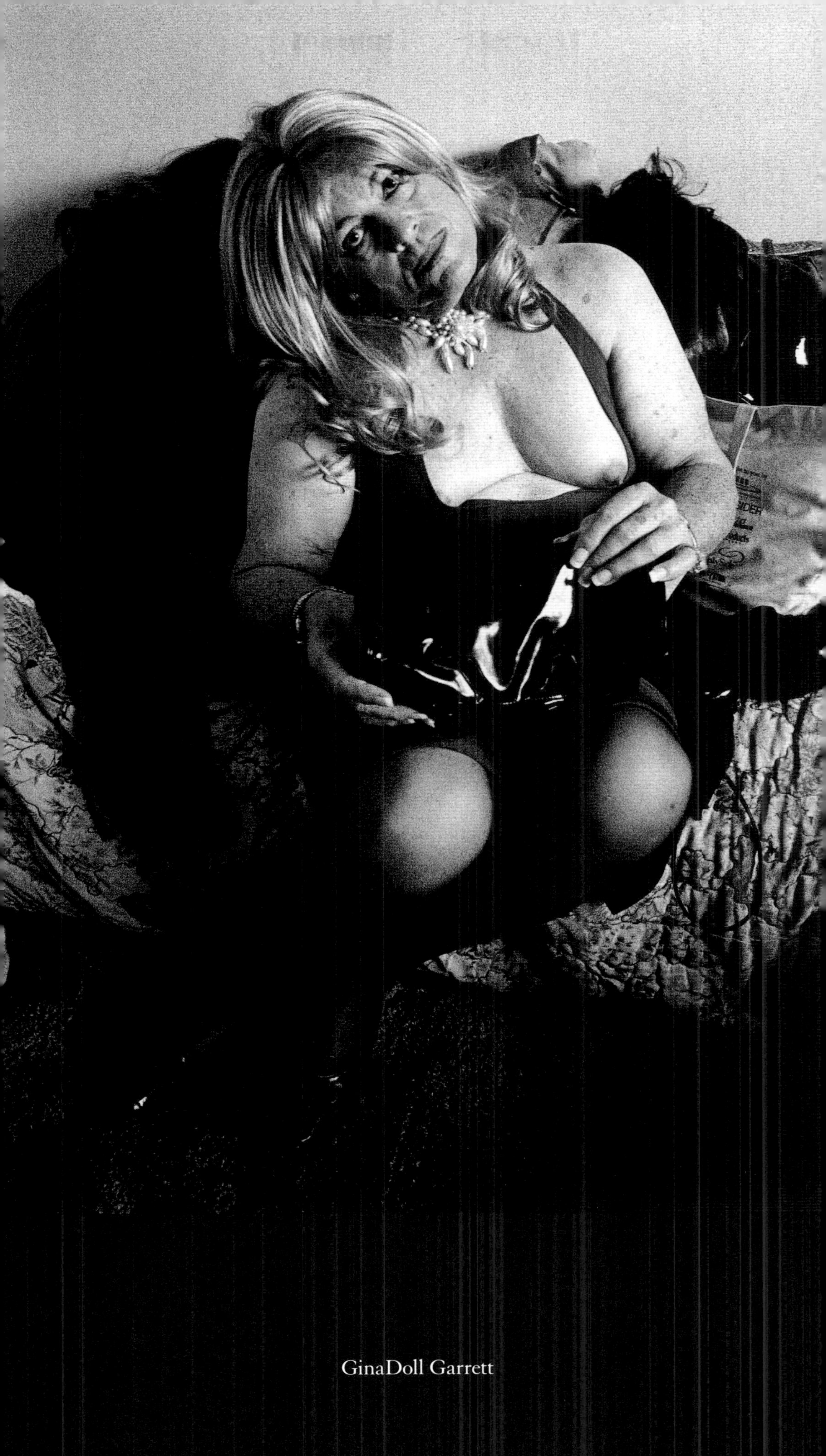

GinaDoll Garrett

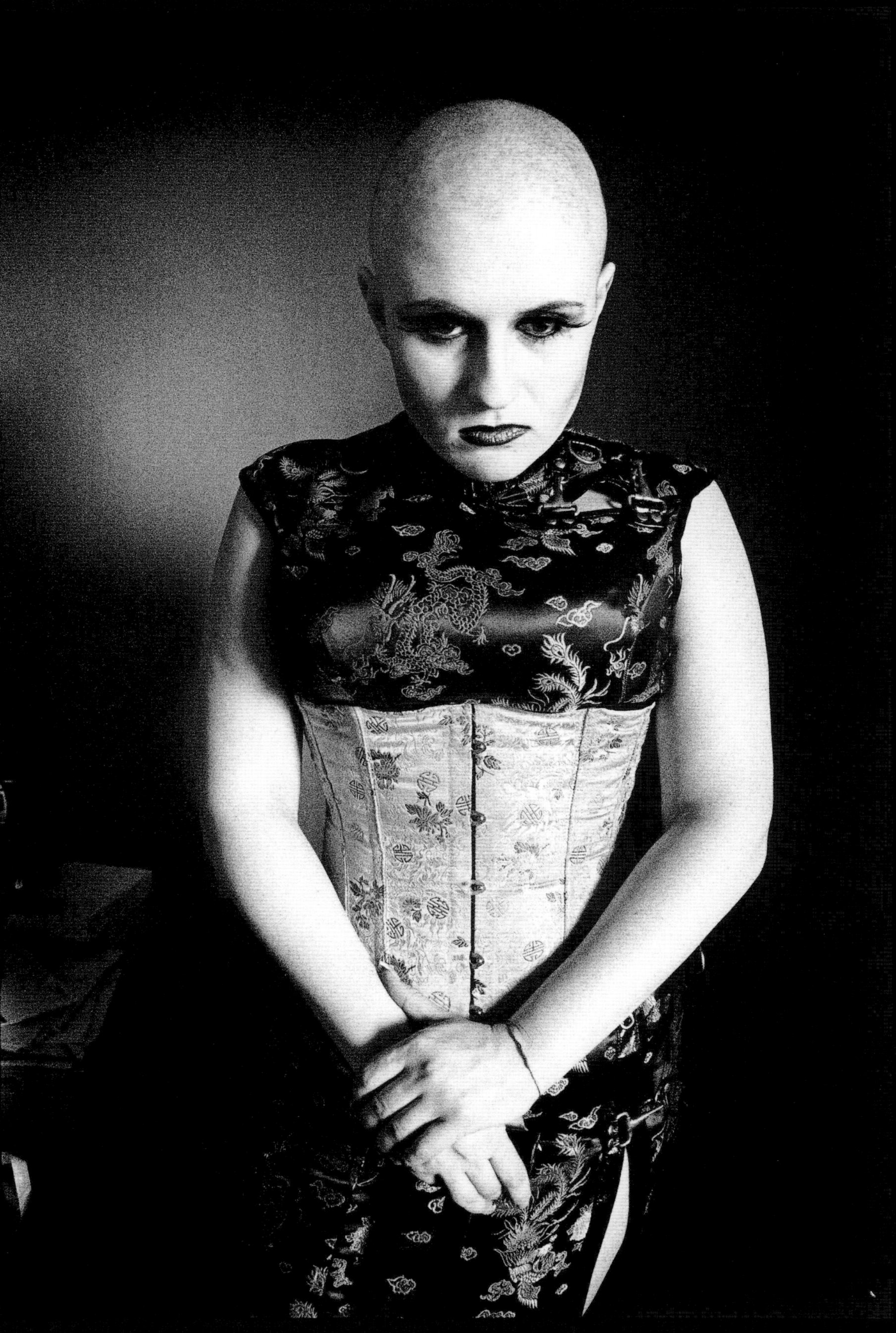

Netochka

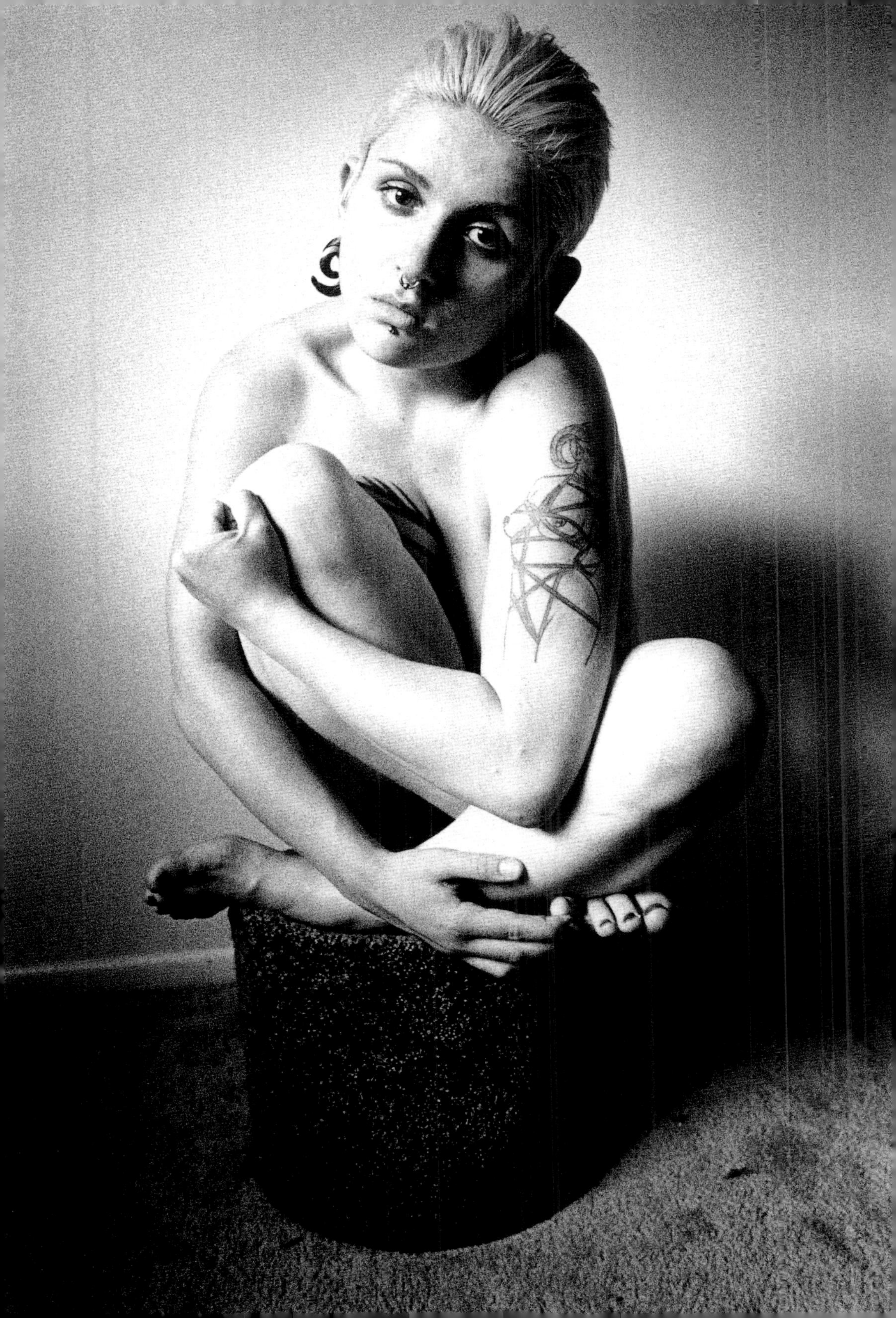

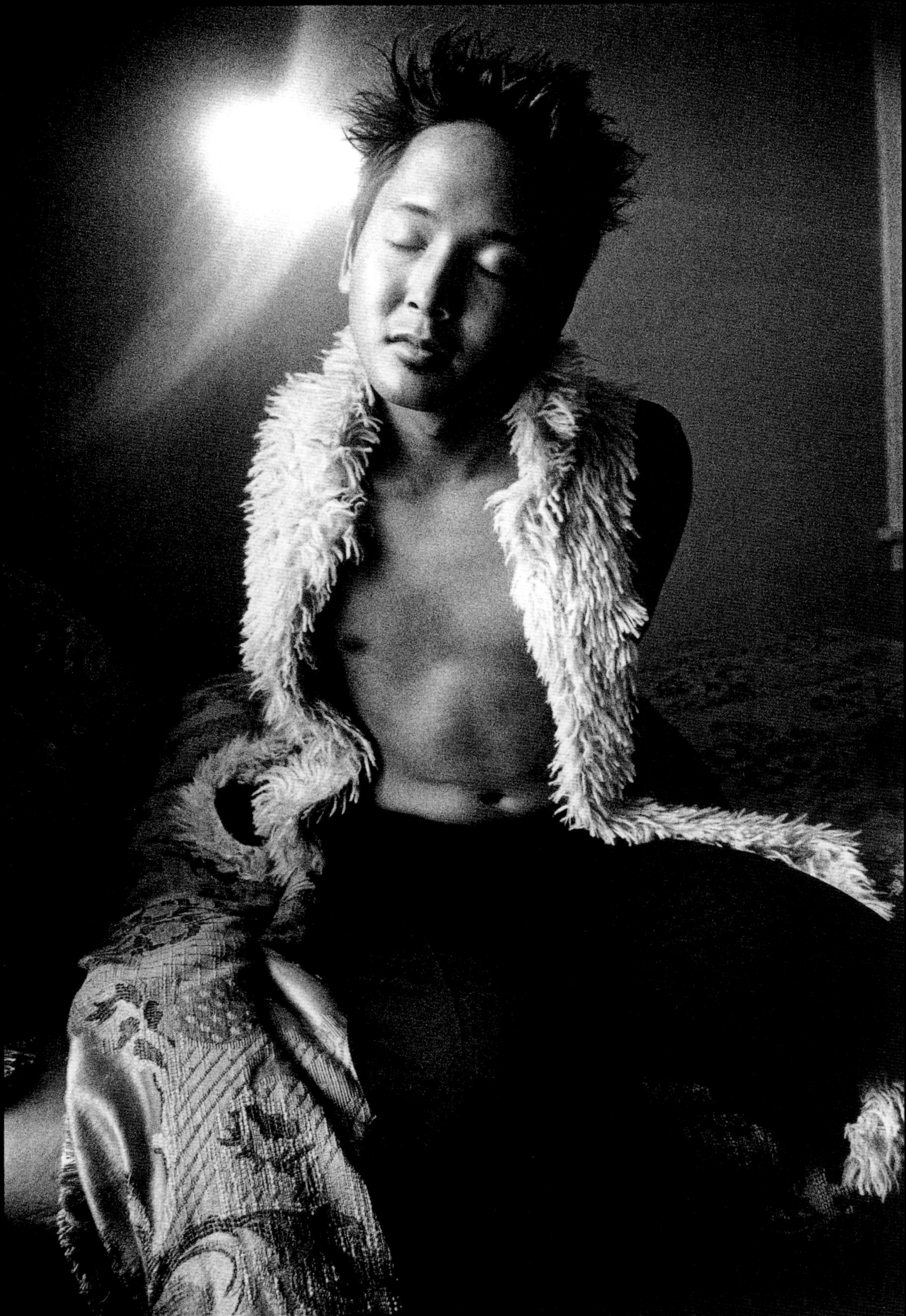

Van Dieu

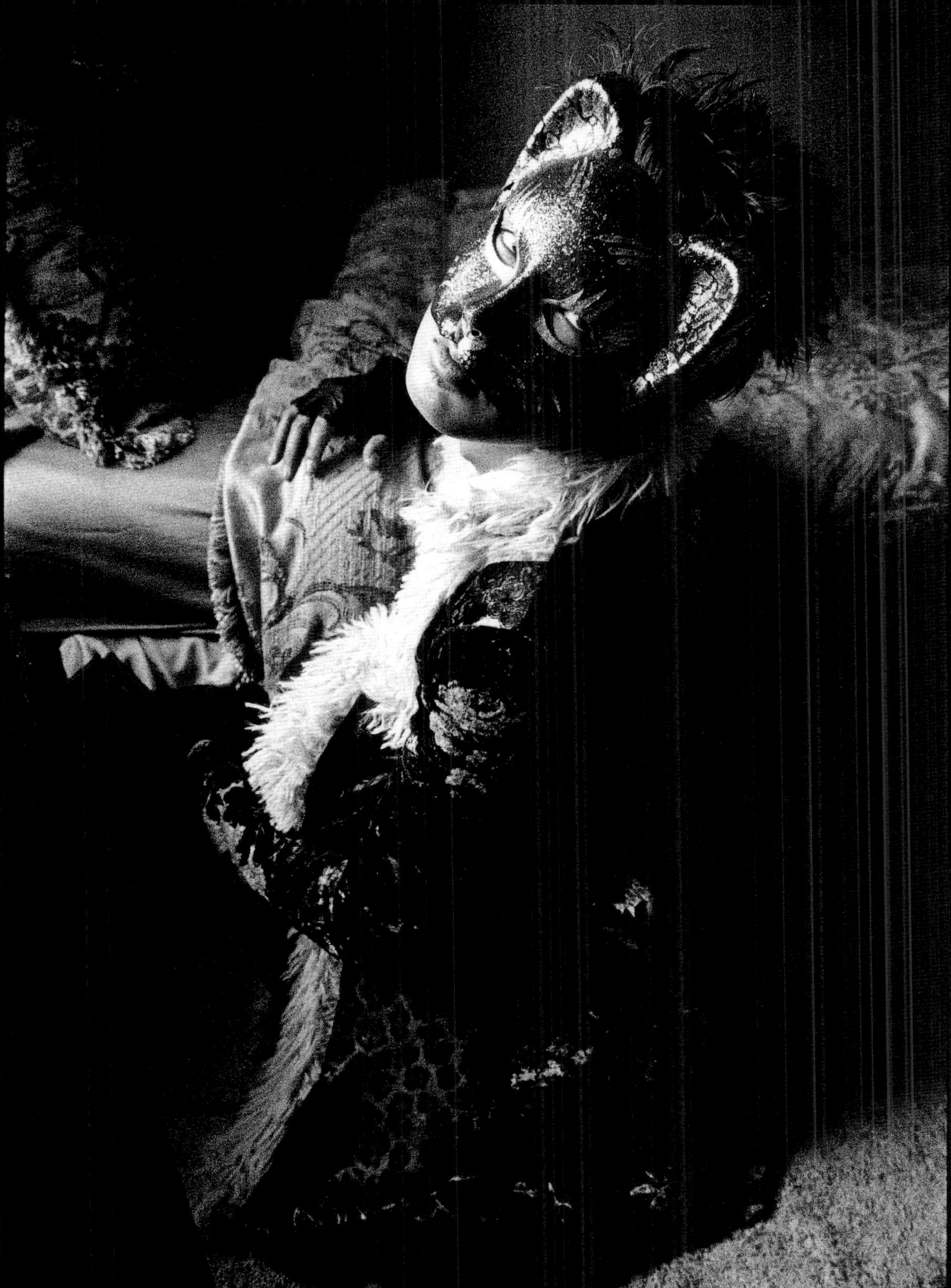

Van Dieu

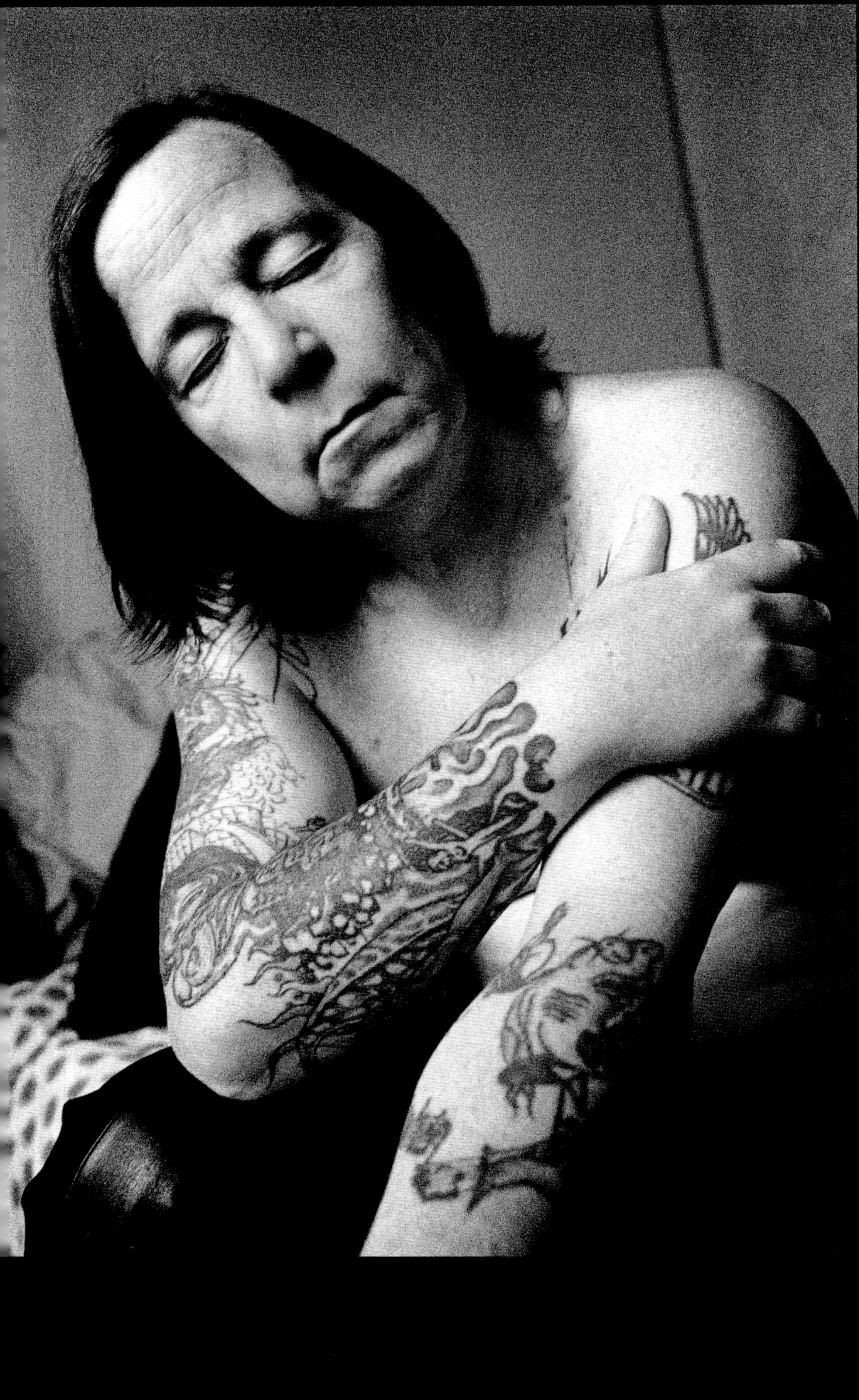

Jimmy

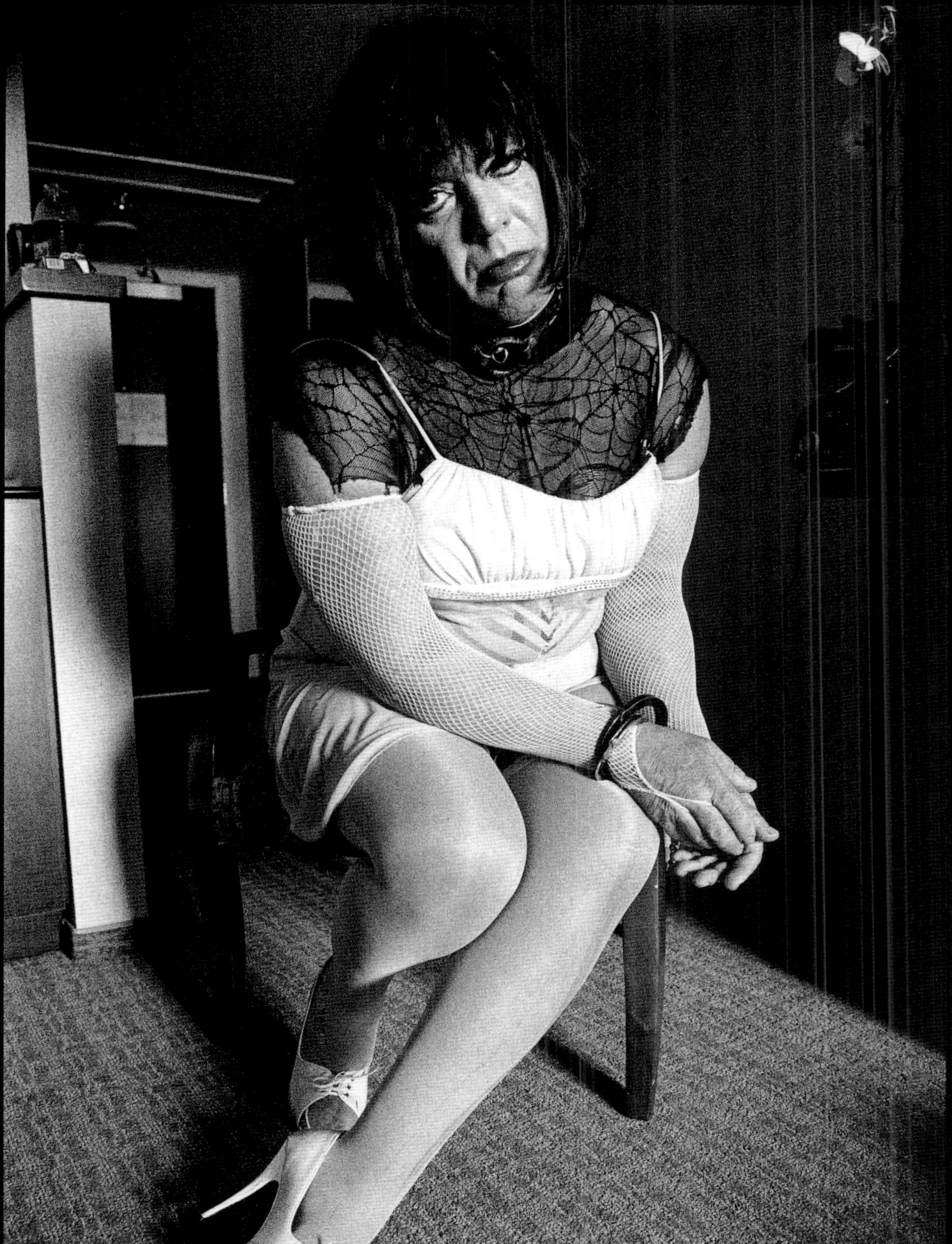

Danna T

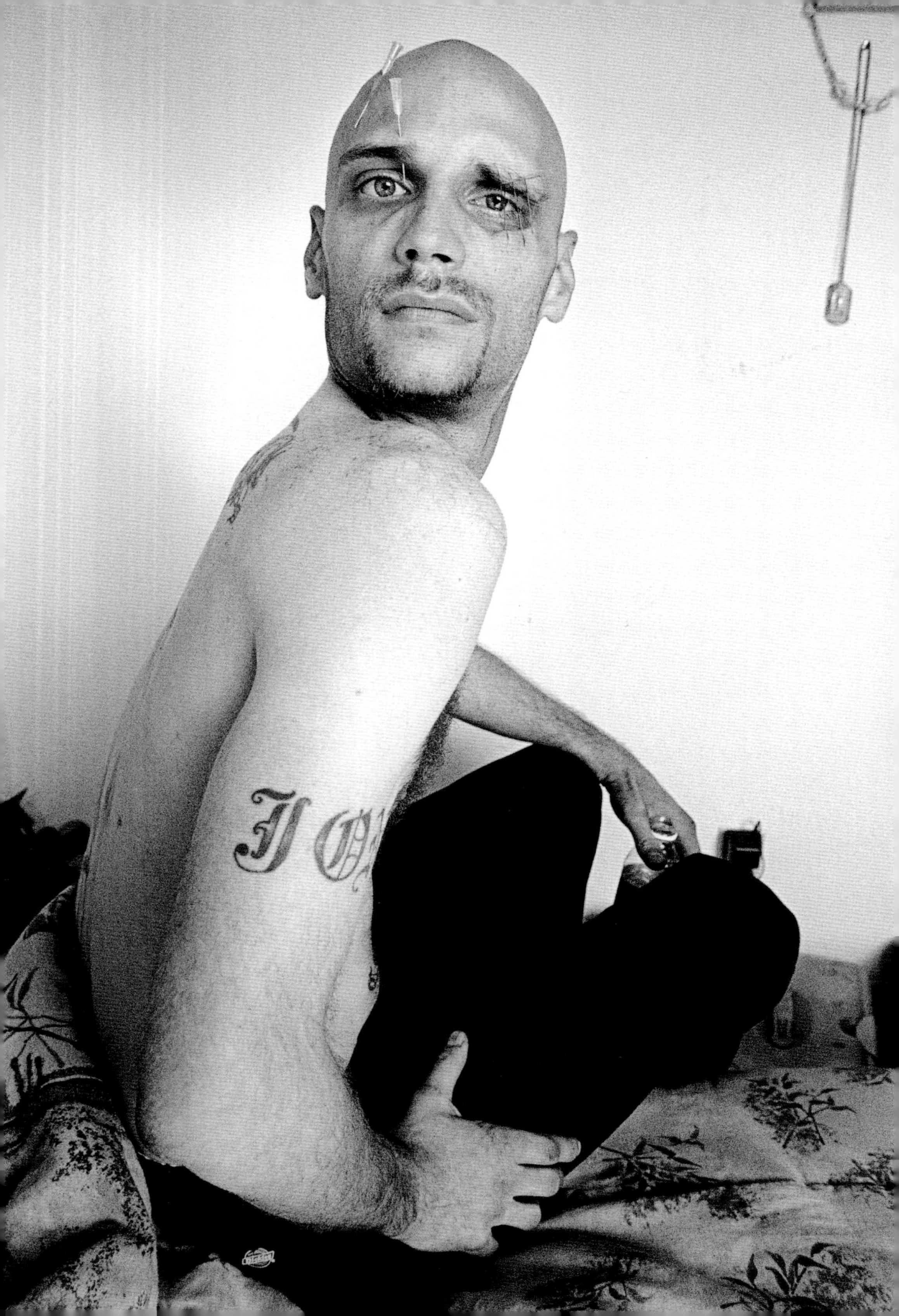

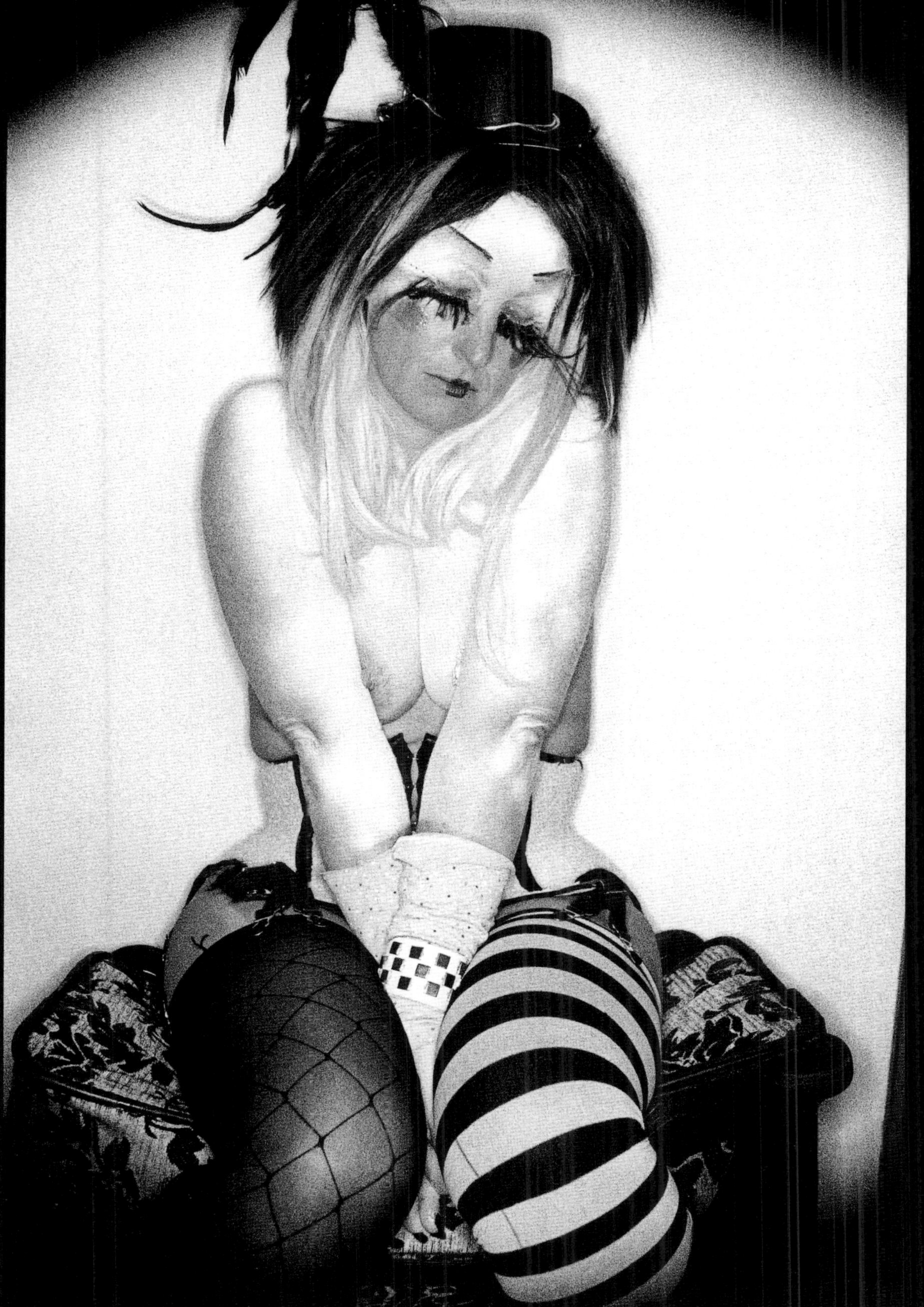

Cari

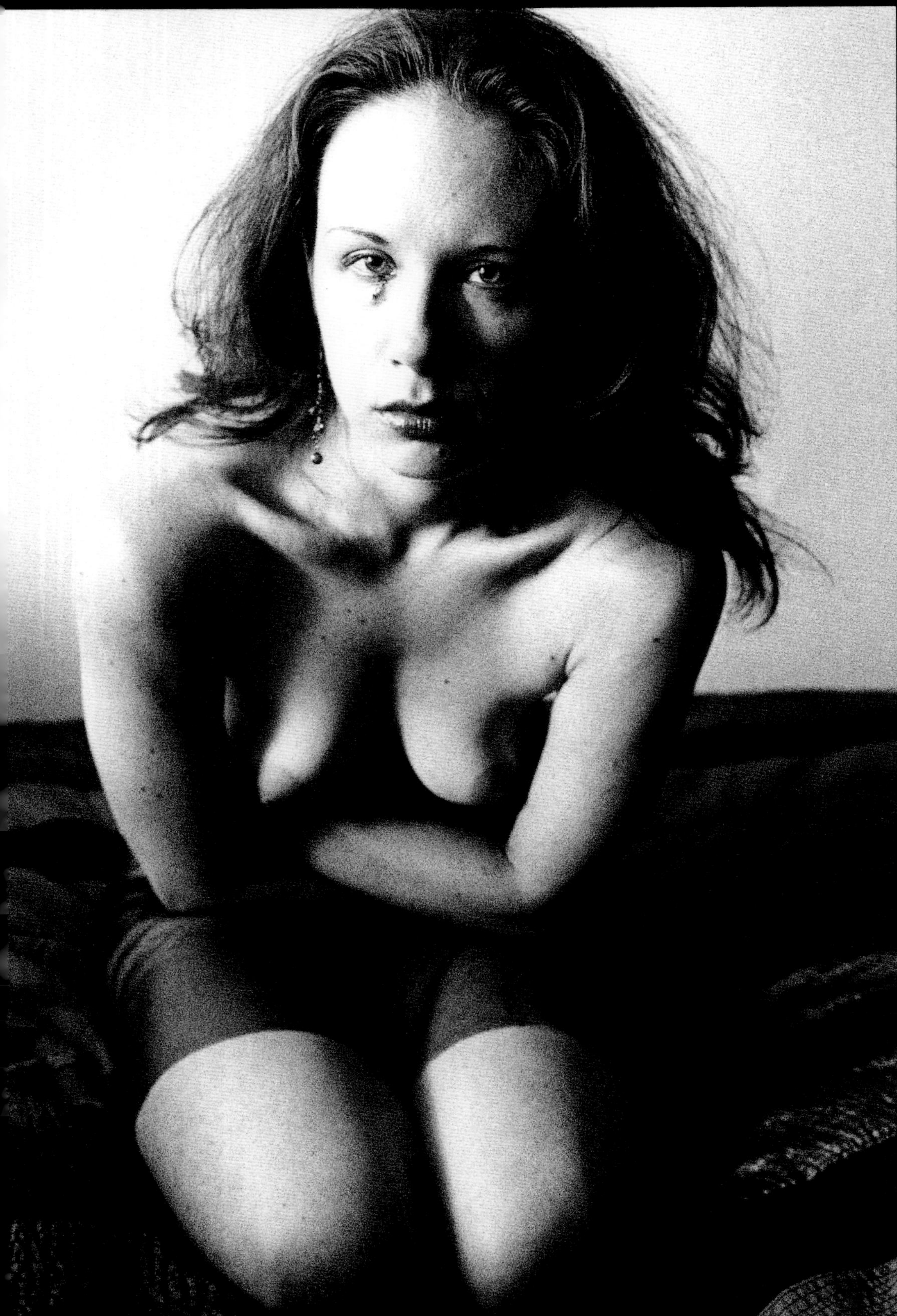

Chas

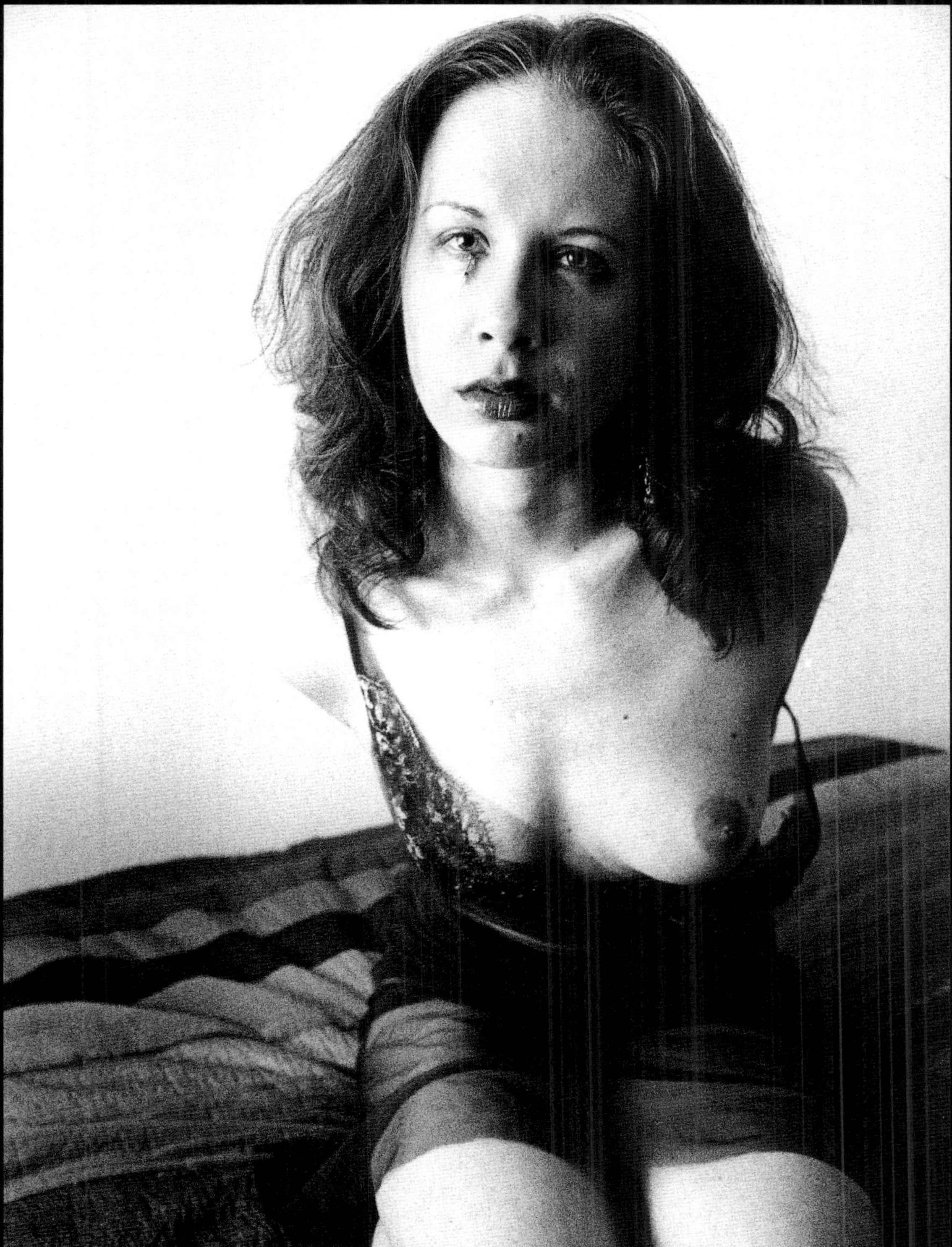

Chas

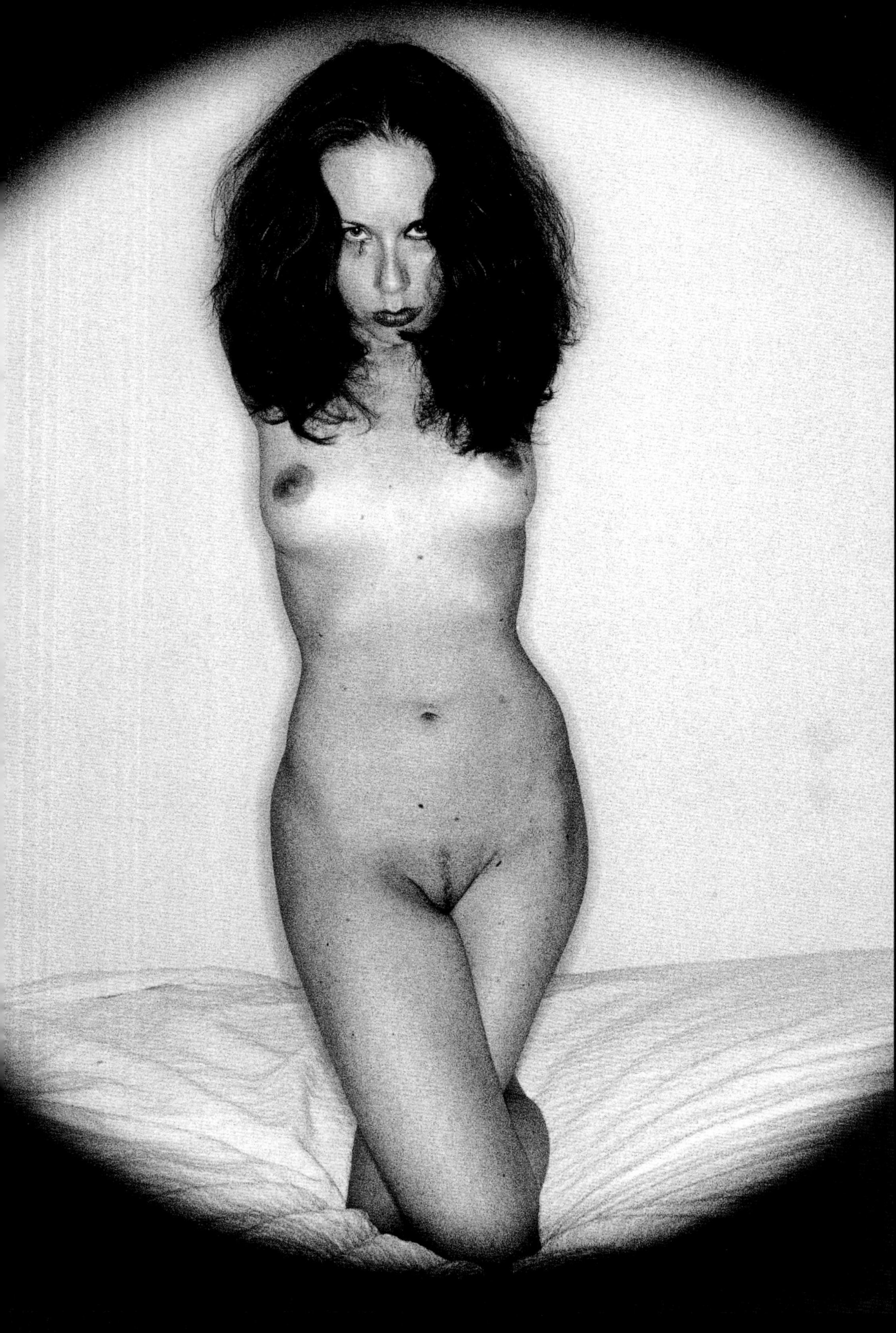

Chas

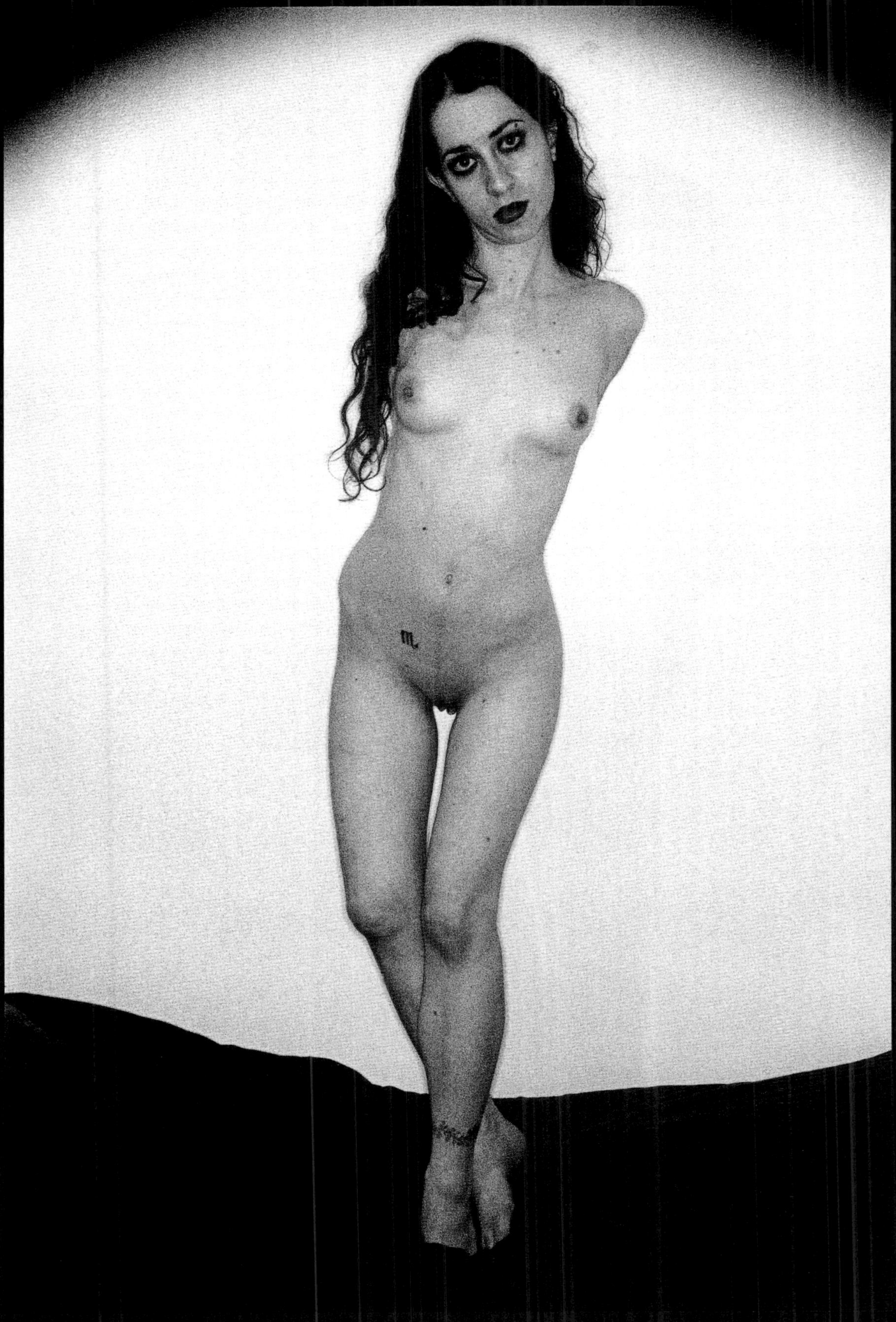

Little Meow · *Overleaf* Little Meow

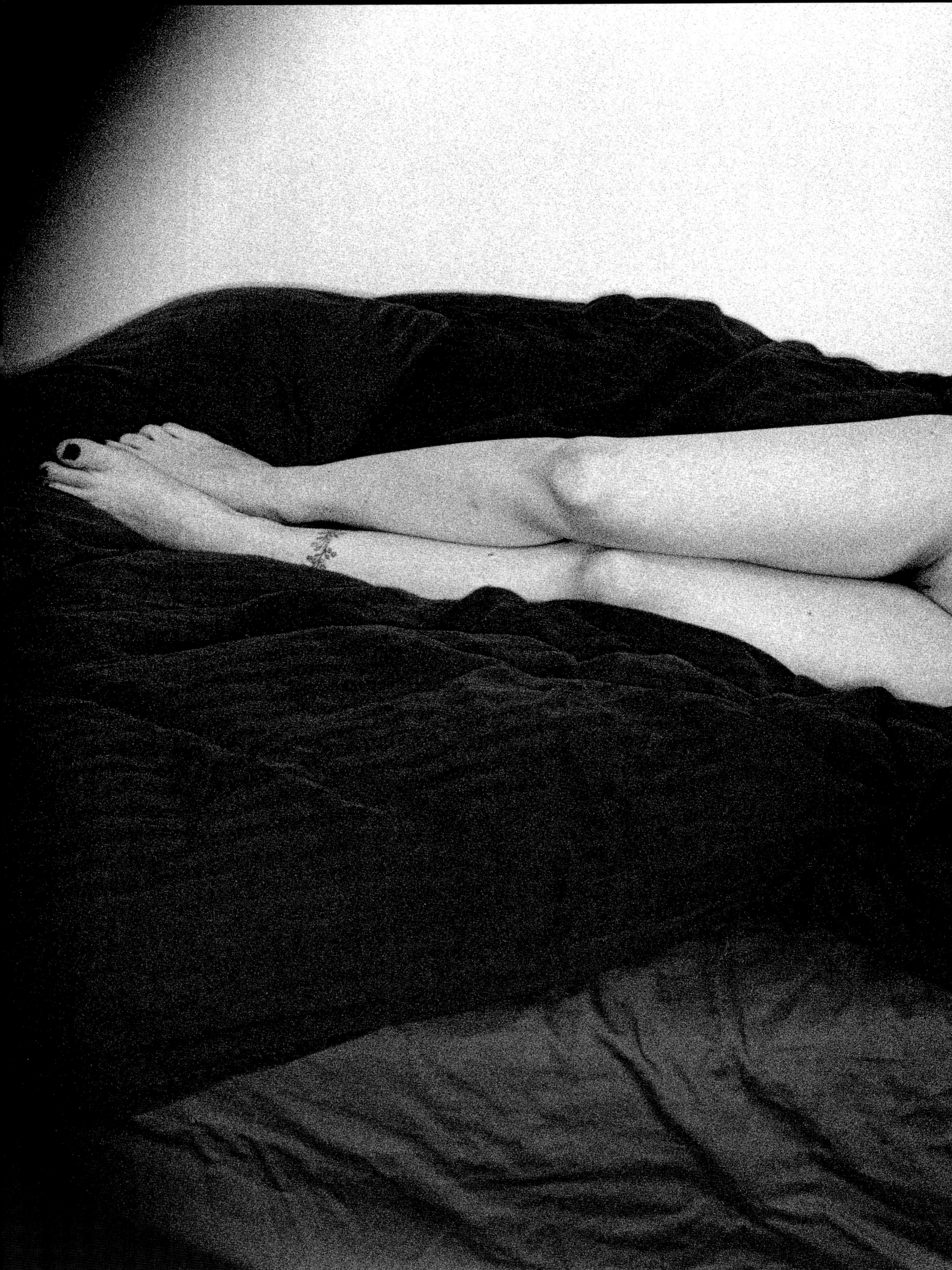

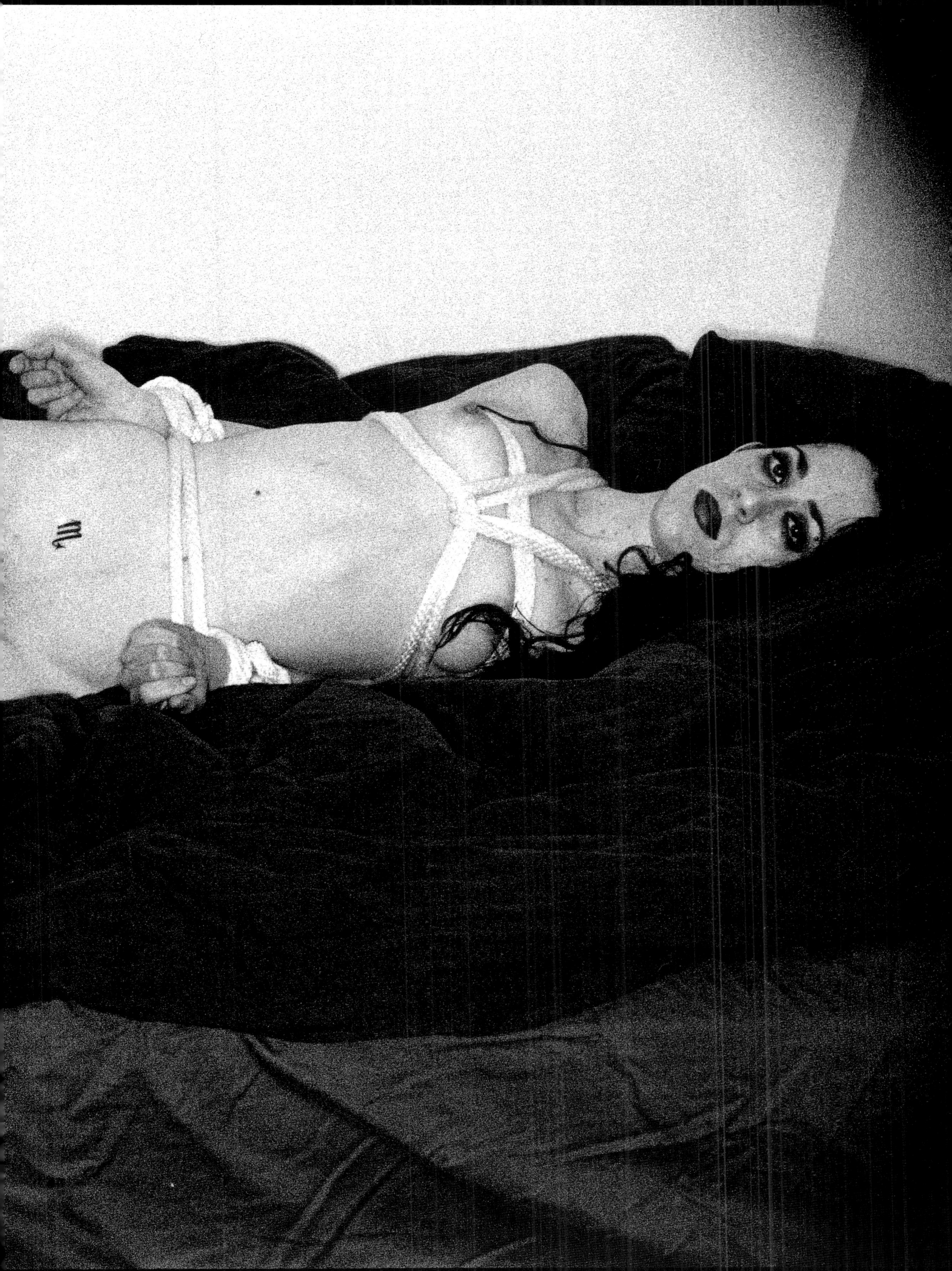

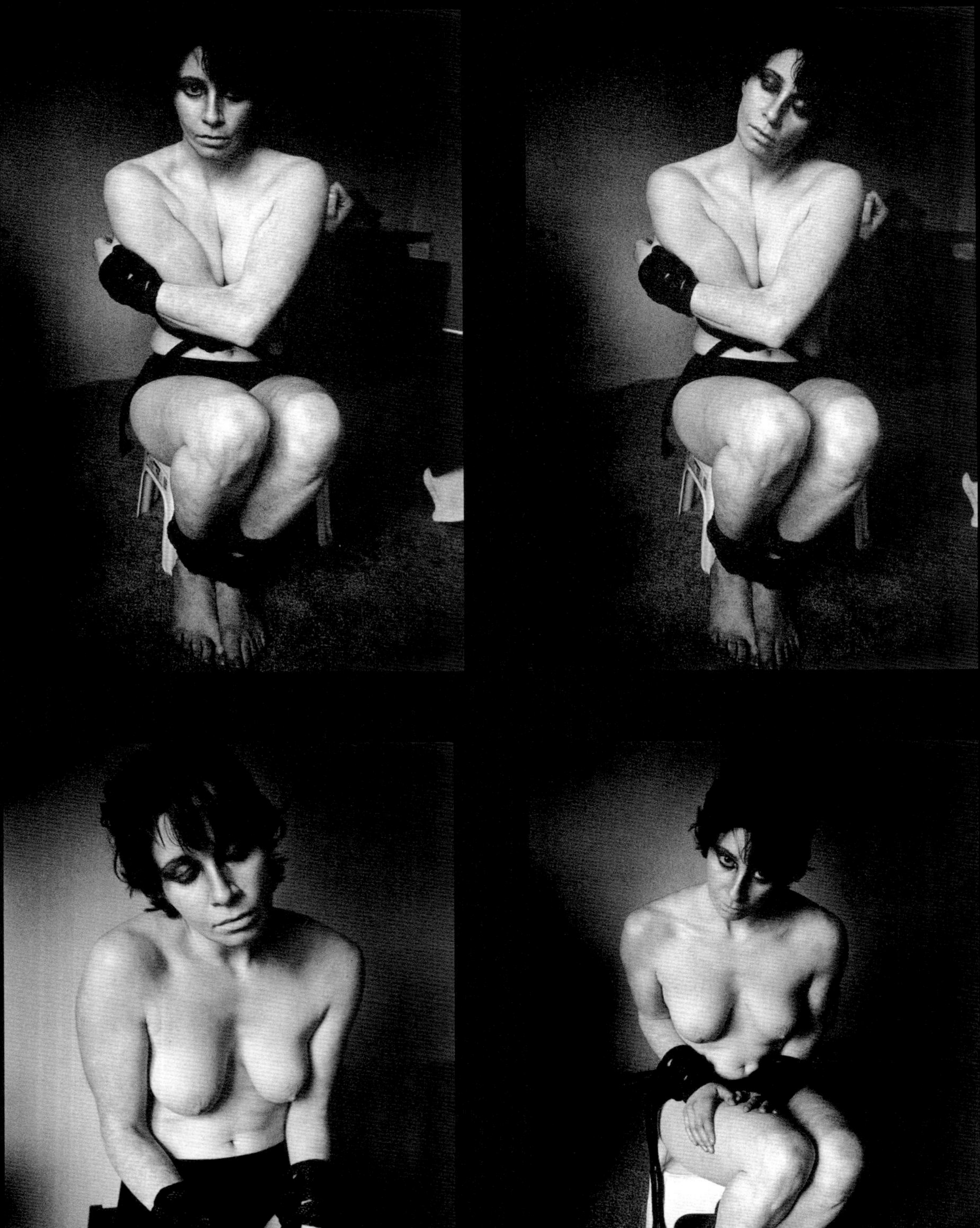

Jordan

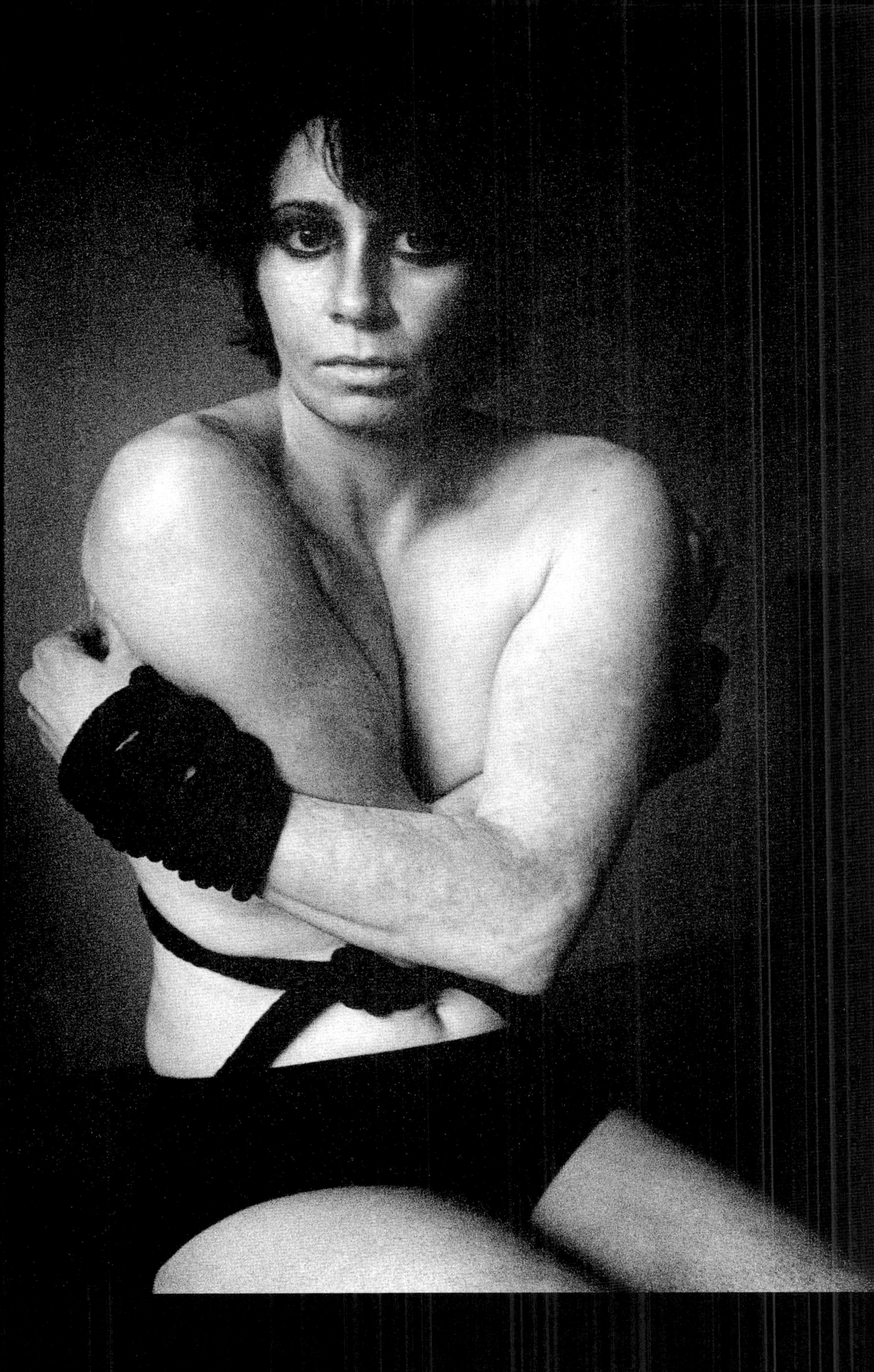

Jordan

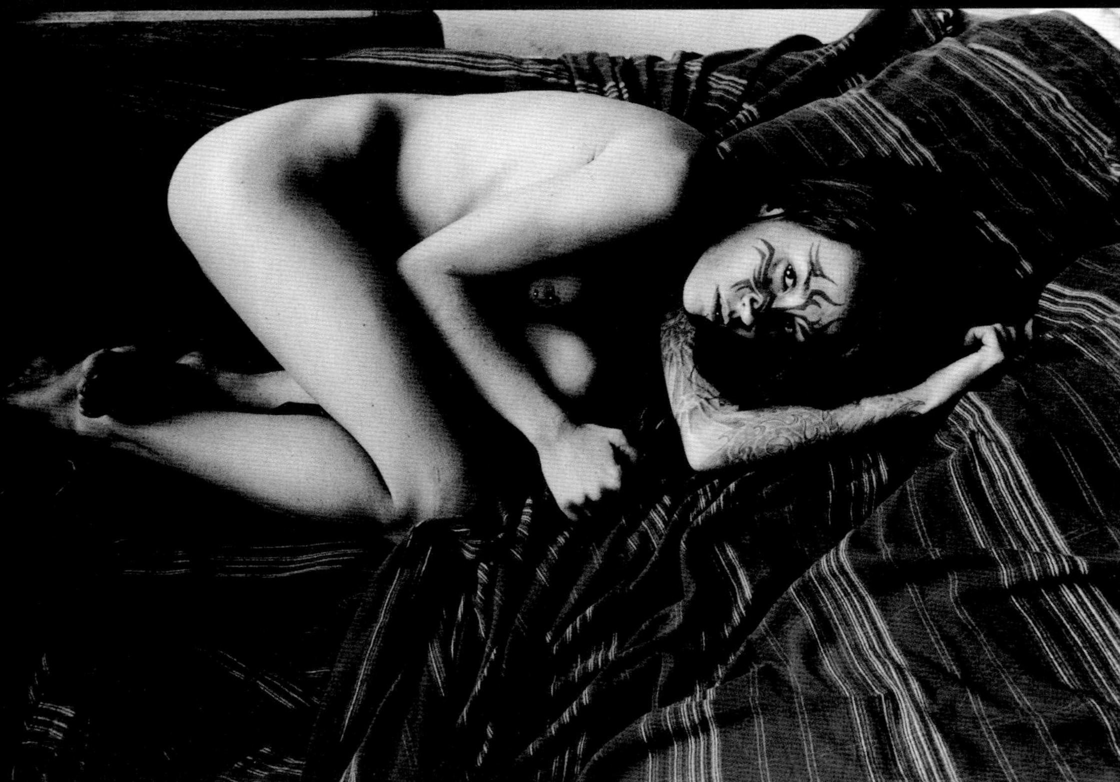

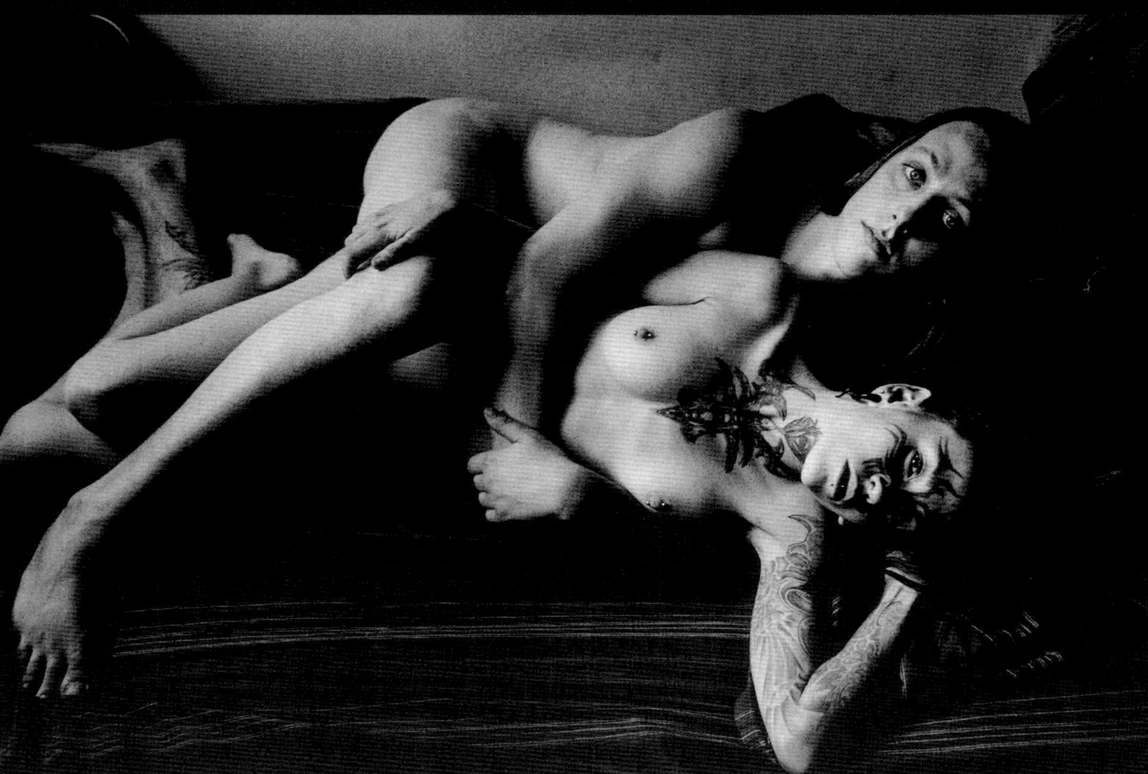

Shannon · Shannon & Dustin

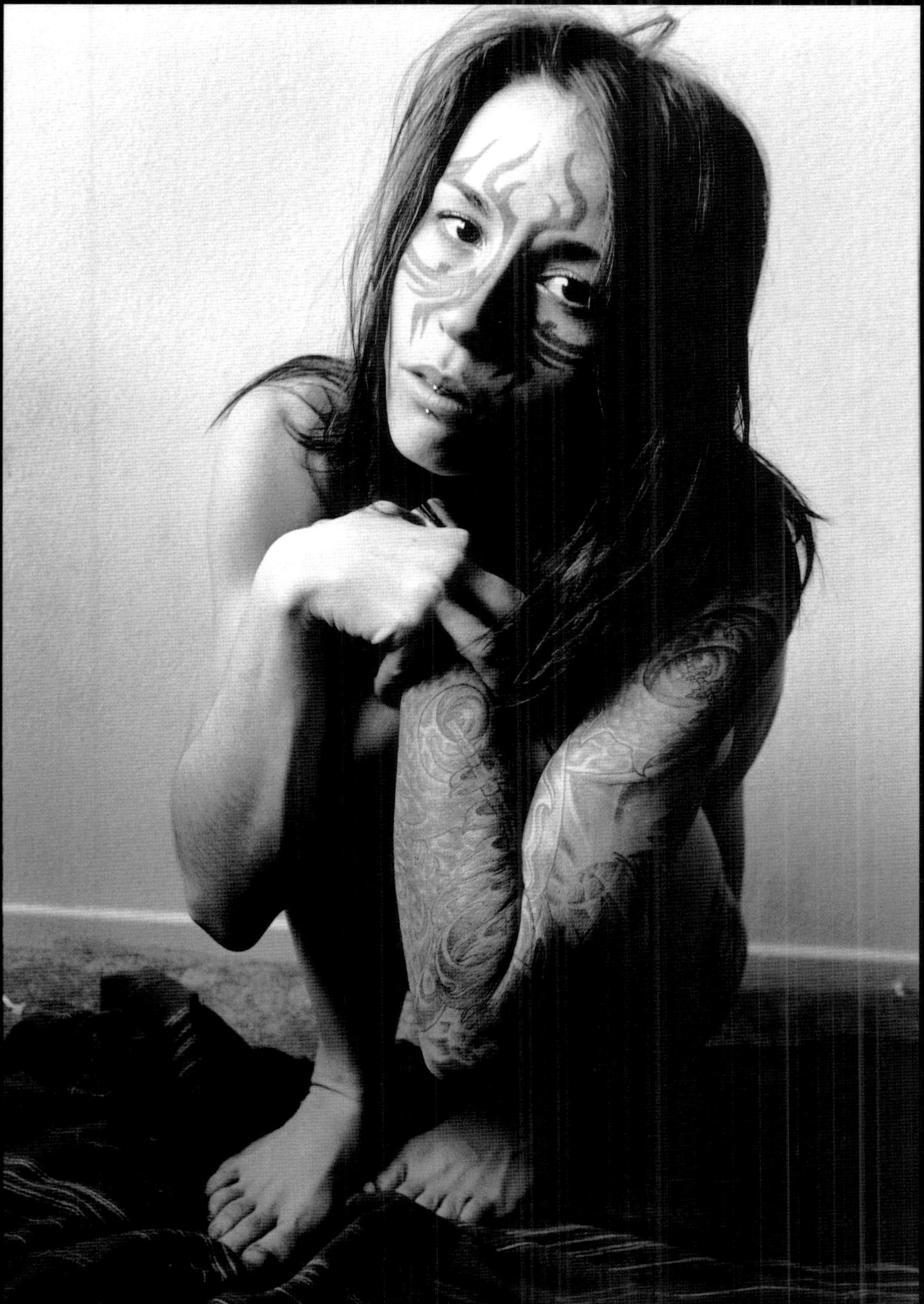

Shannon

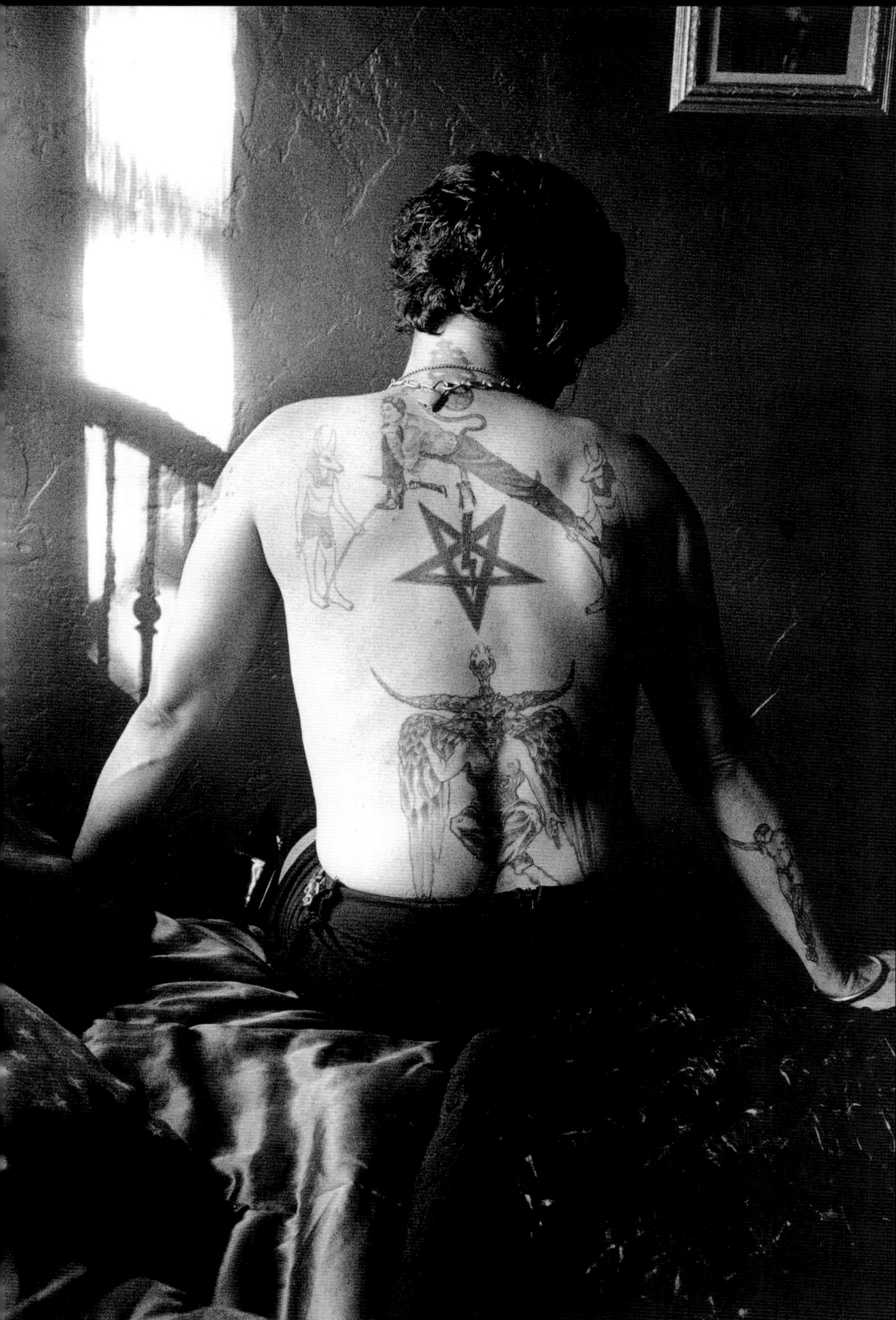

Sal

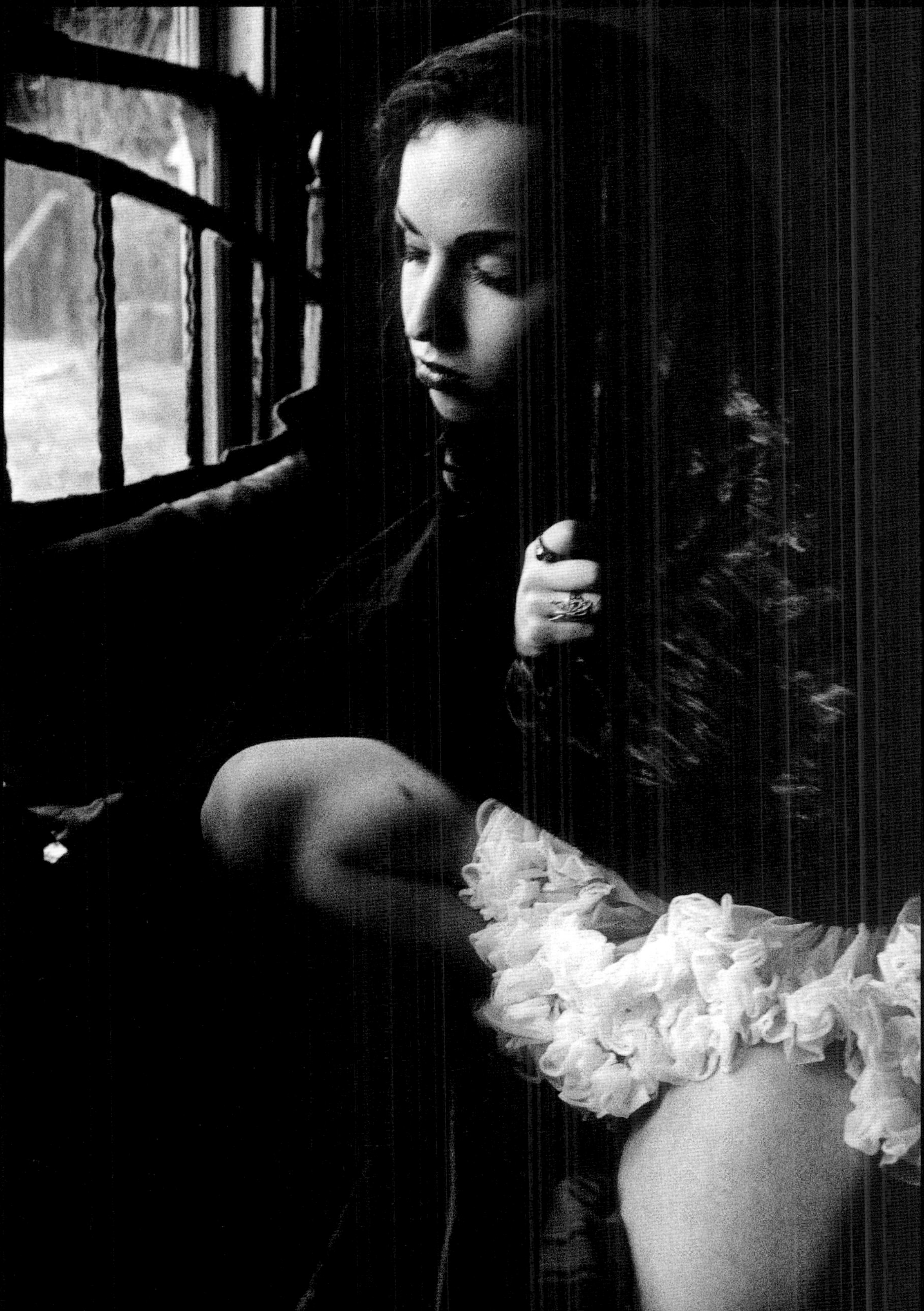

Rachael

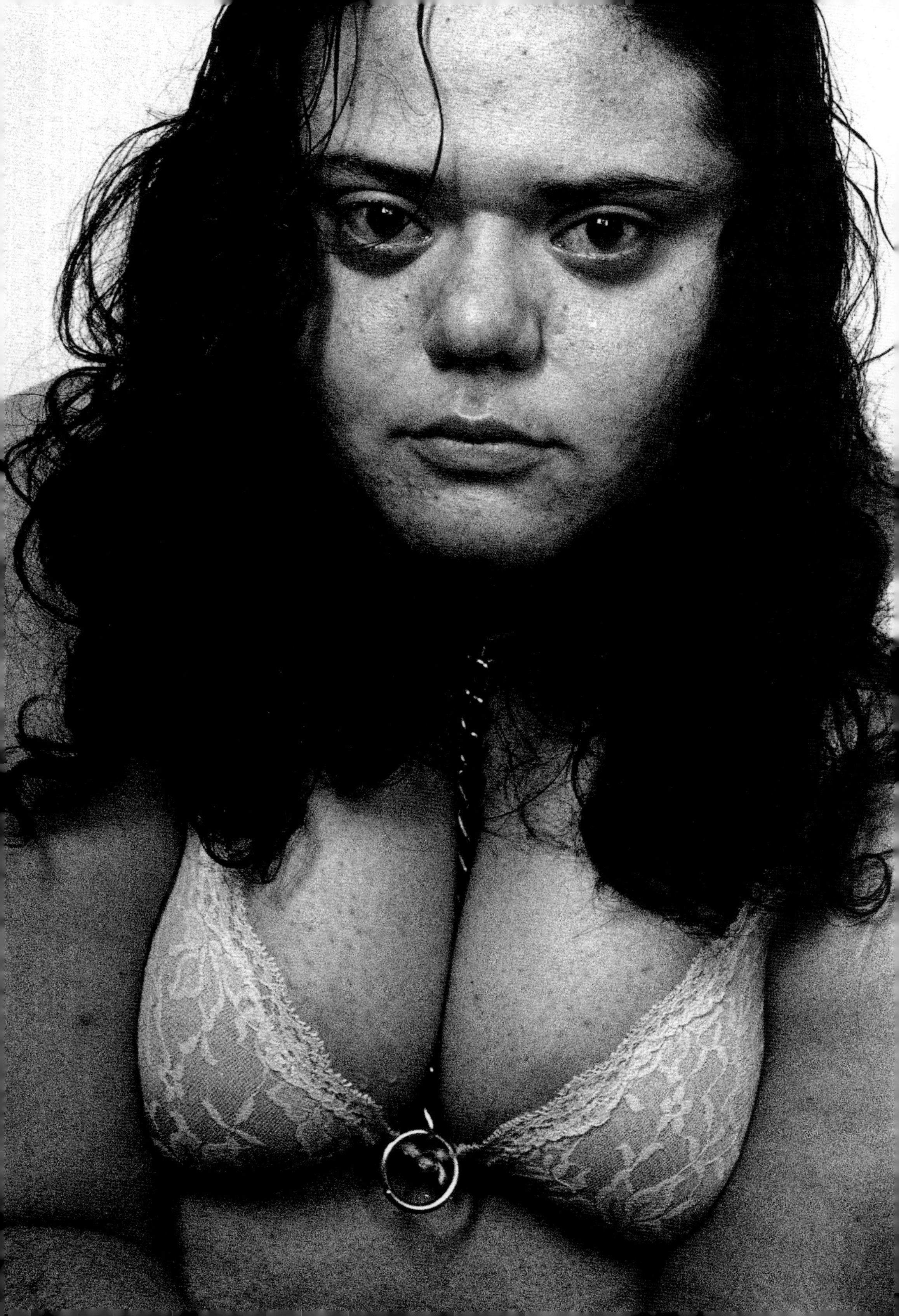

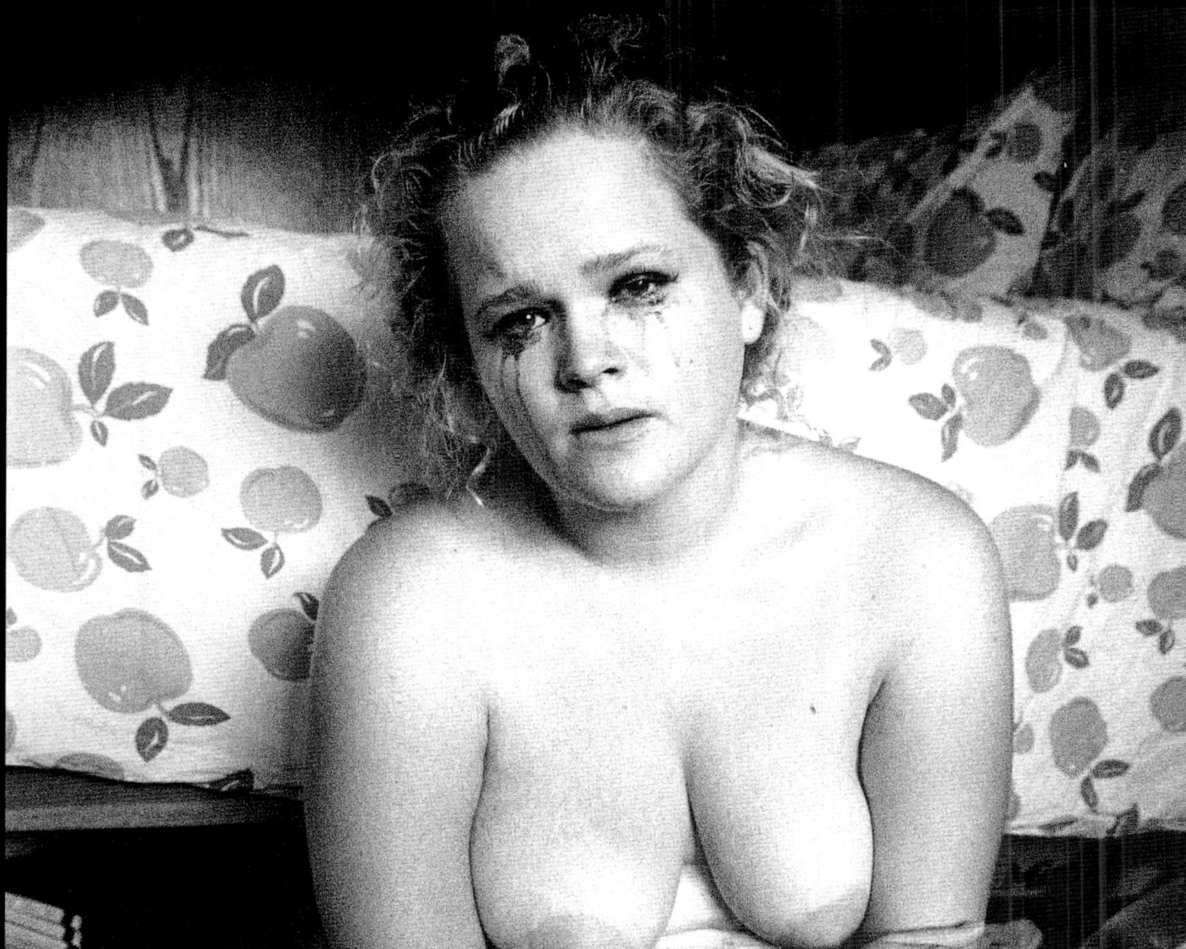

Whitney

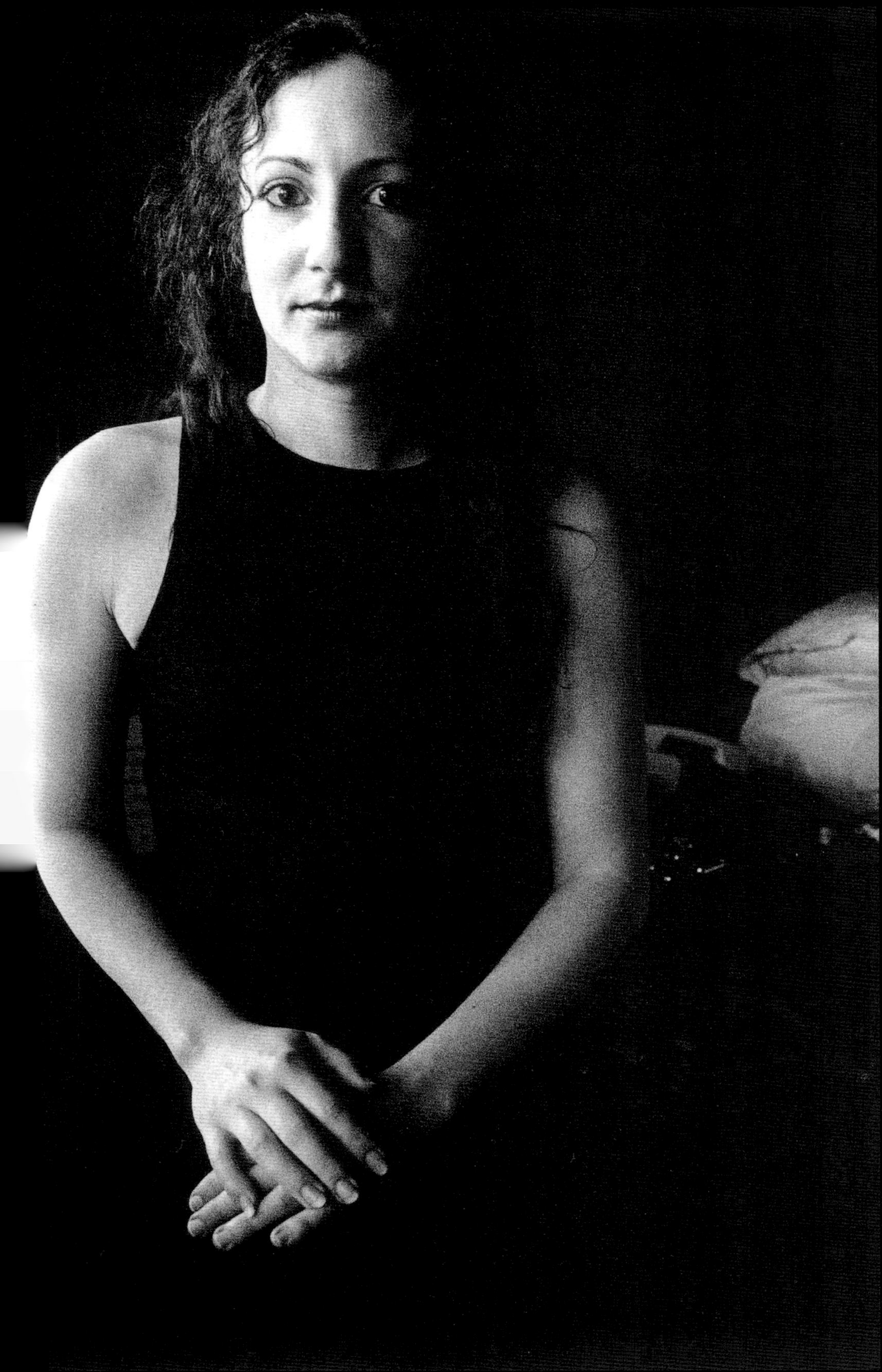

Joseph

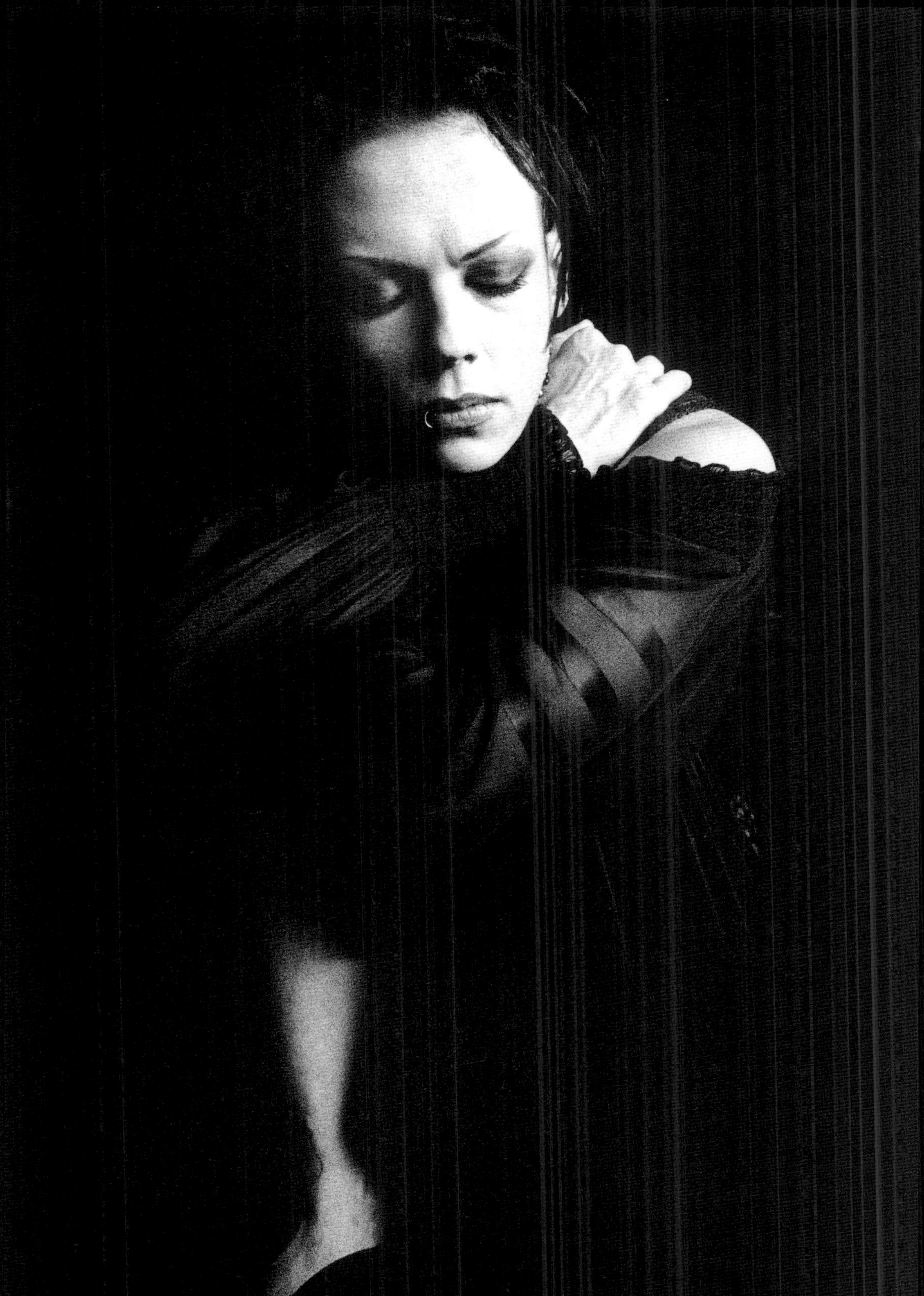

Pia

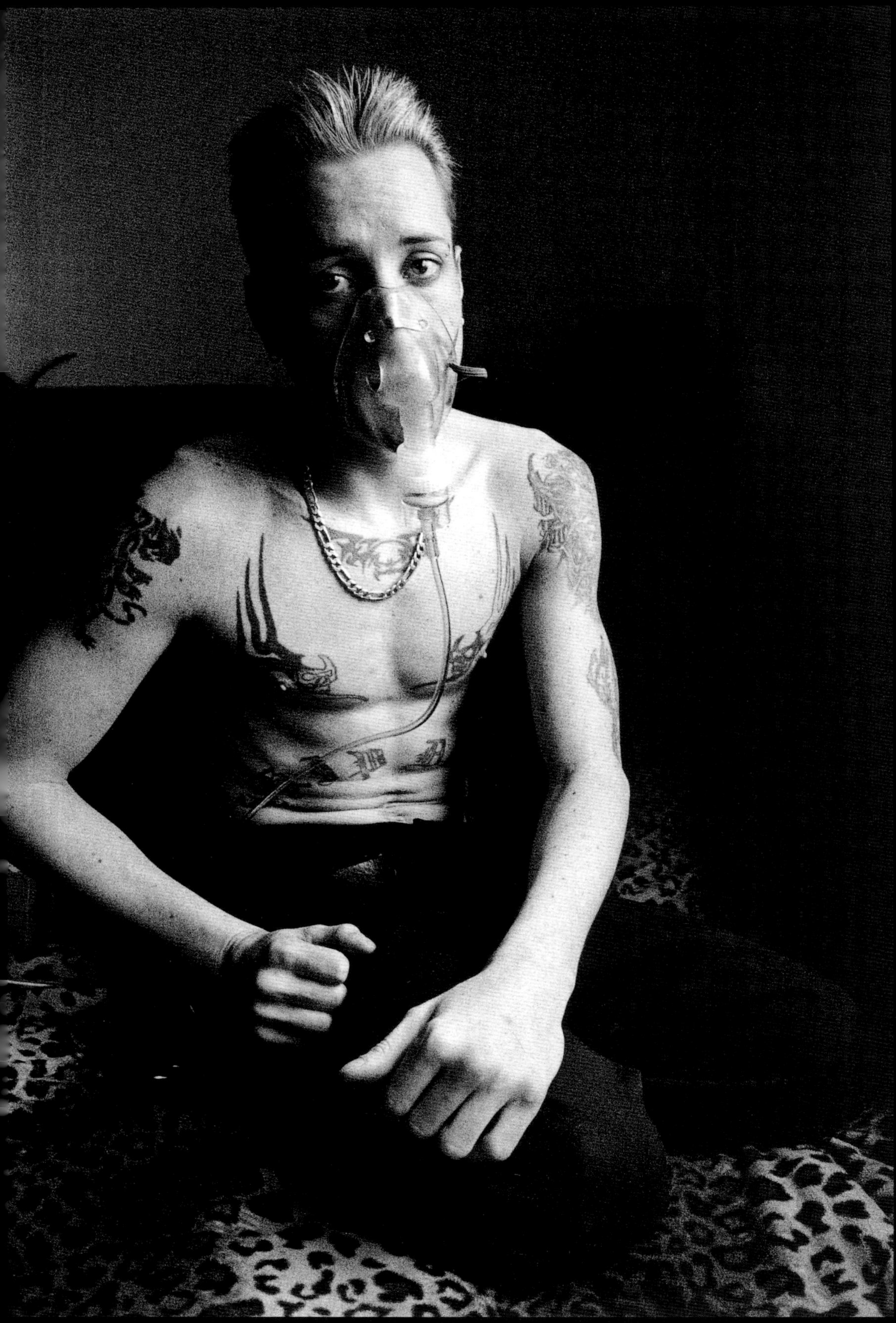

Skipdog

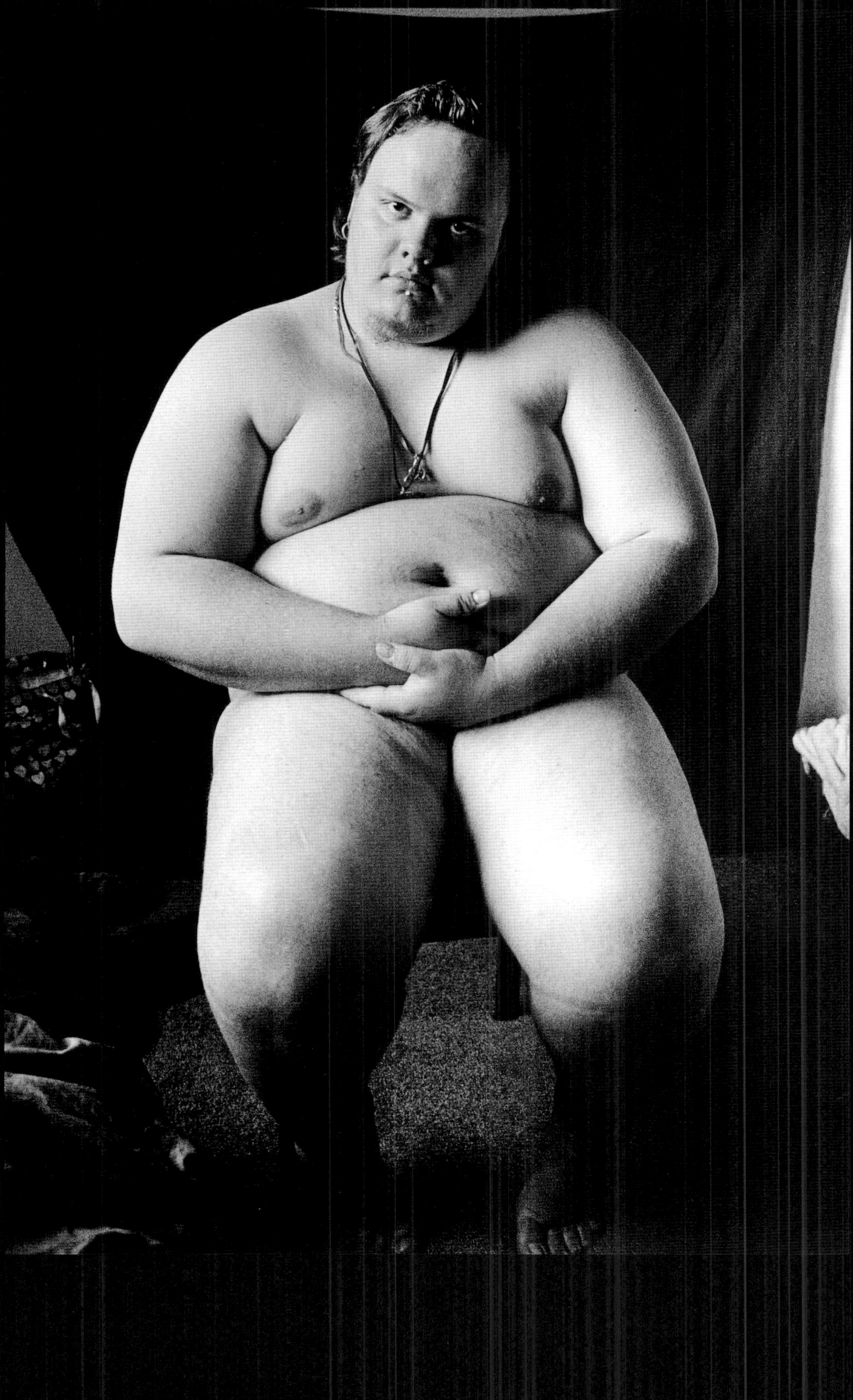

Scotty

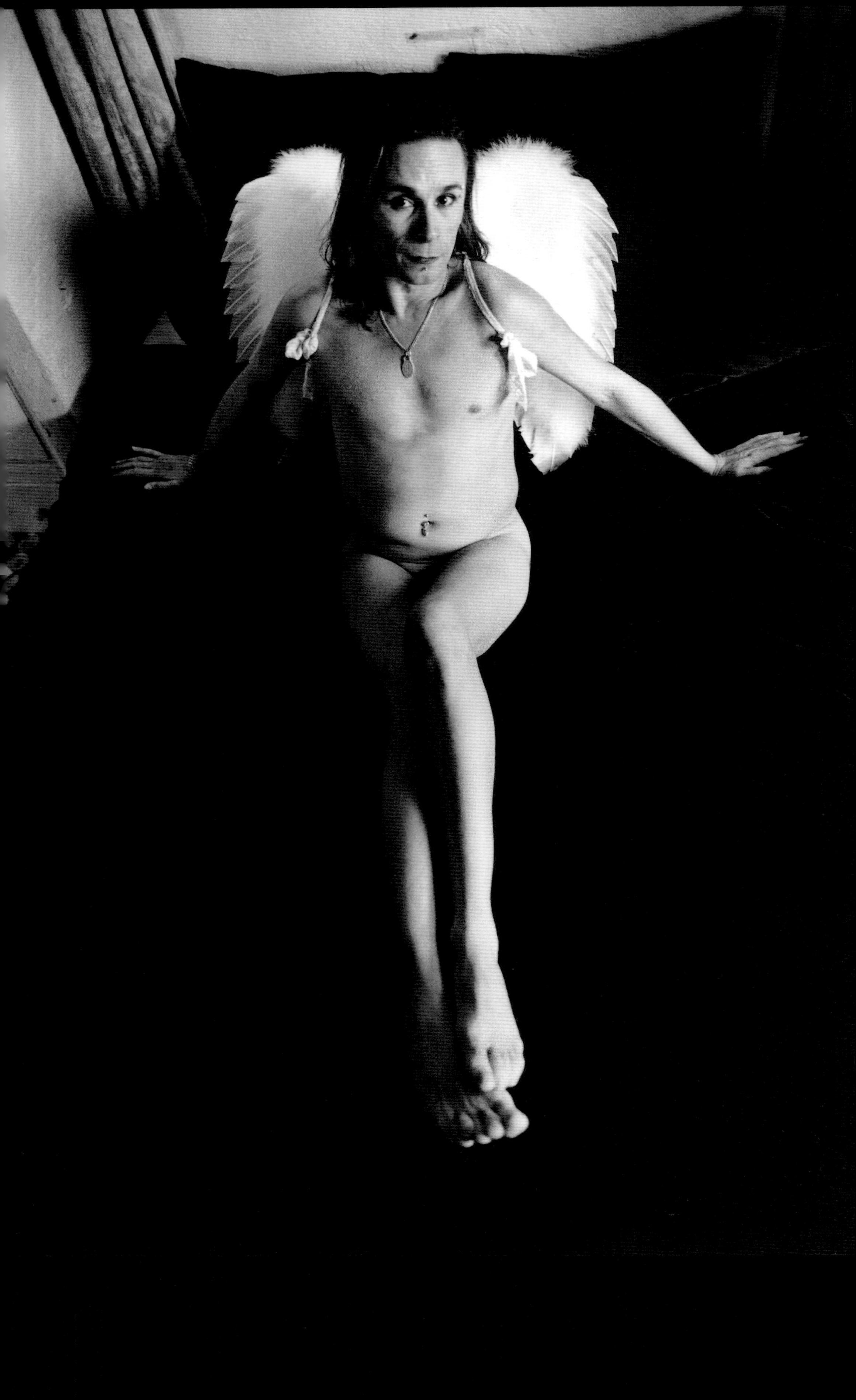

Ashley

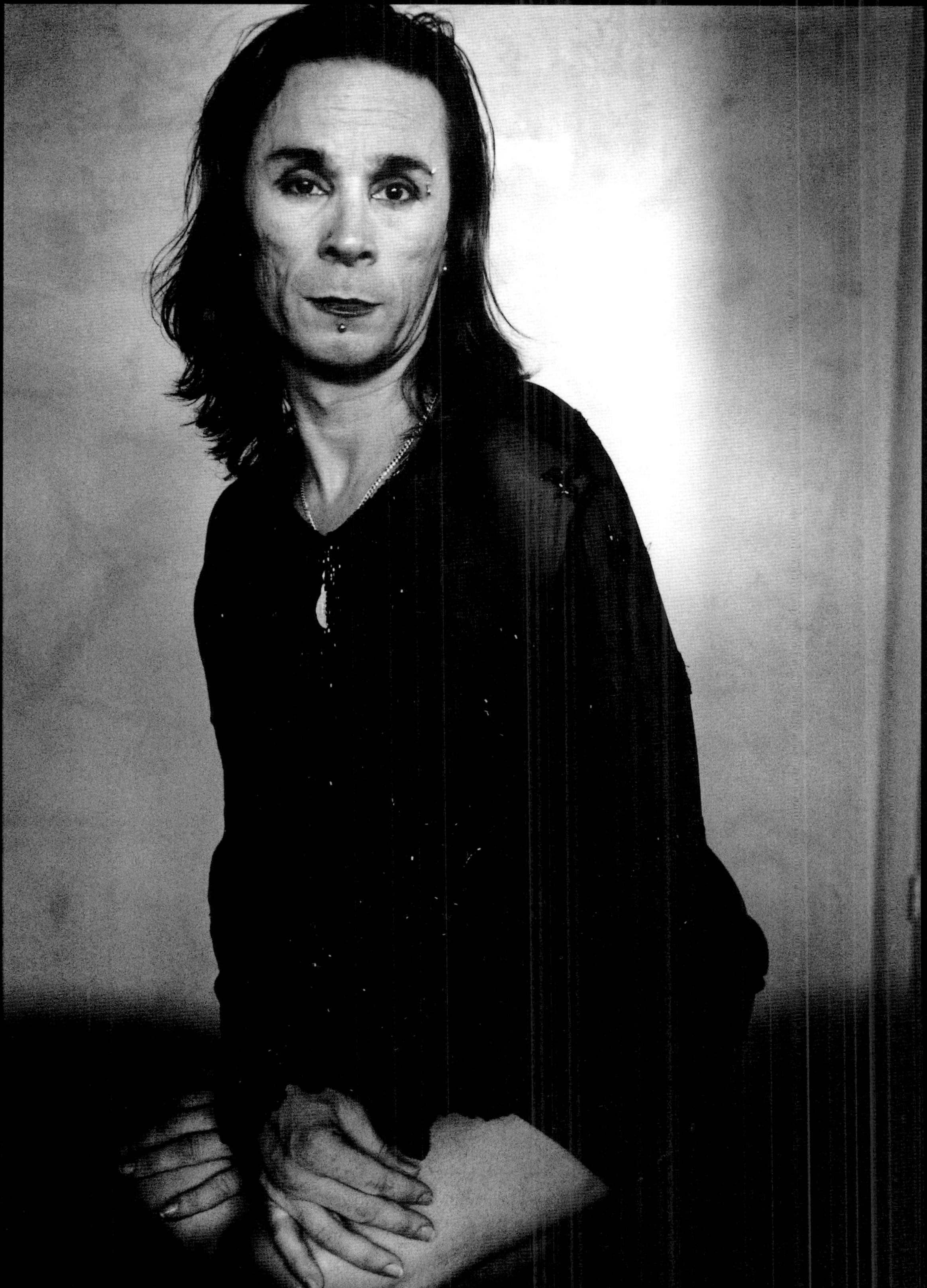

Ashley

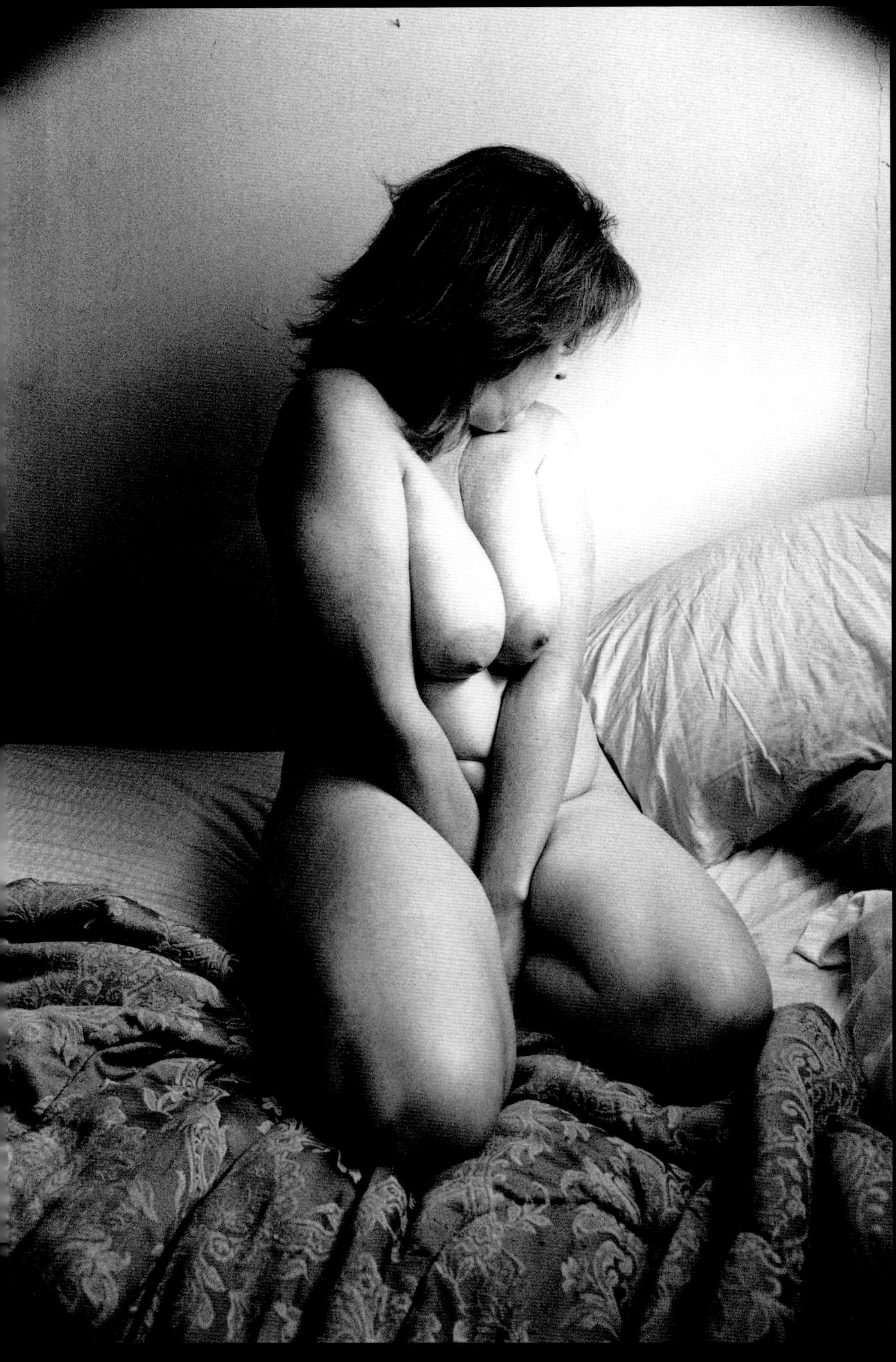

Jeanne Marie

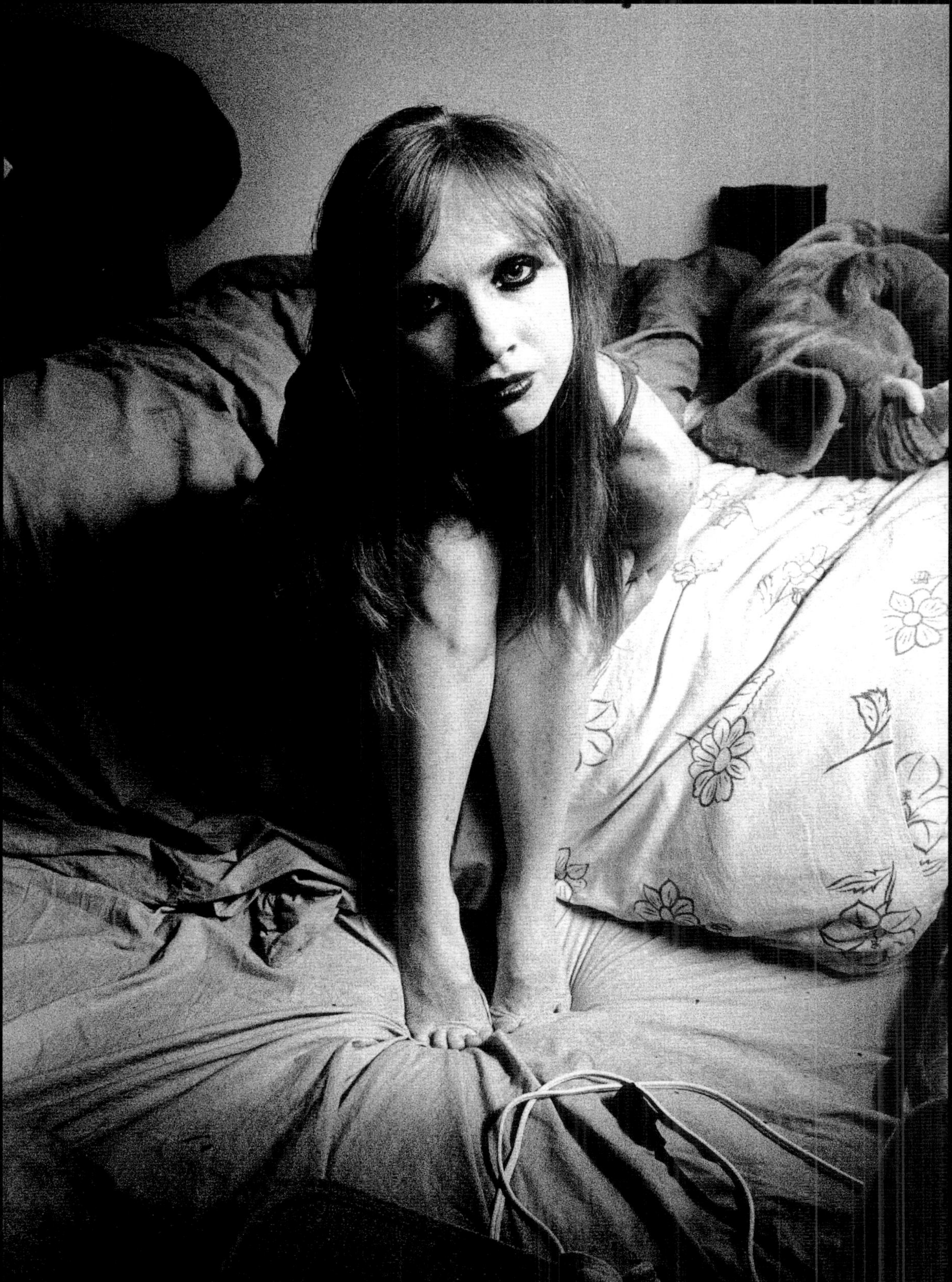

Sarryh

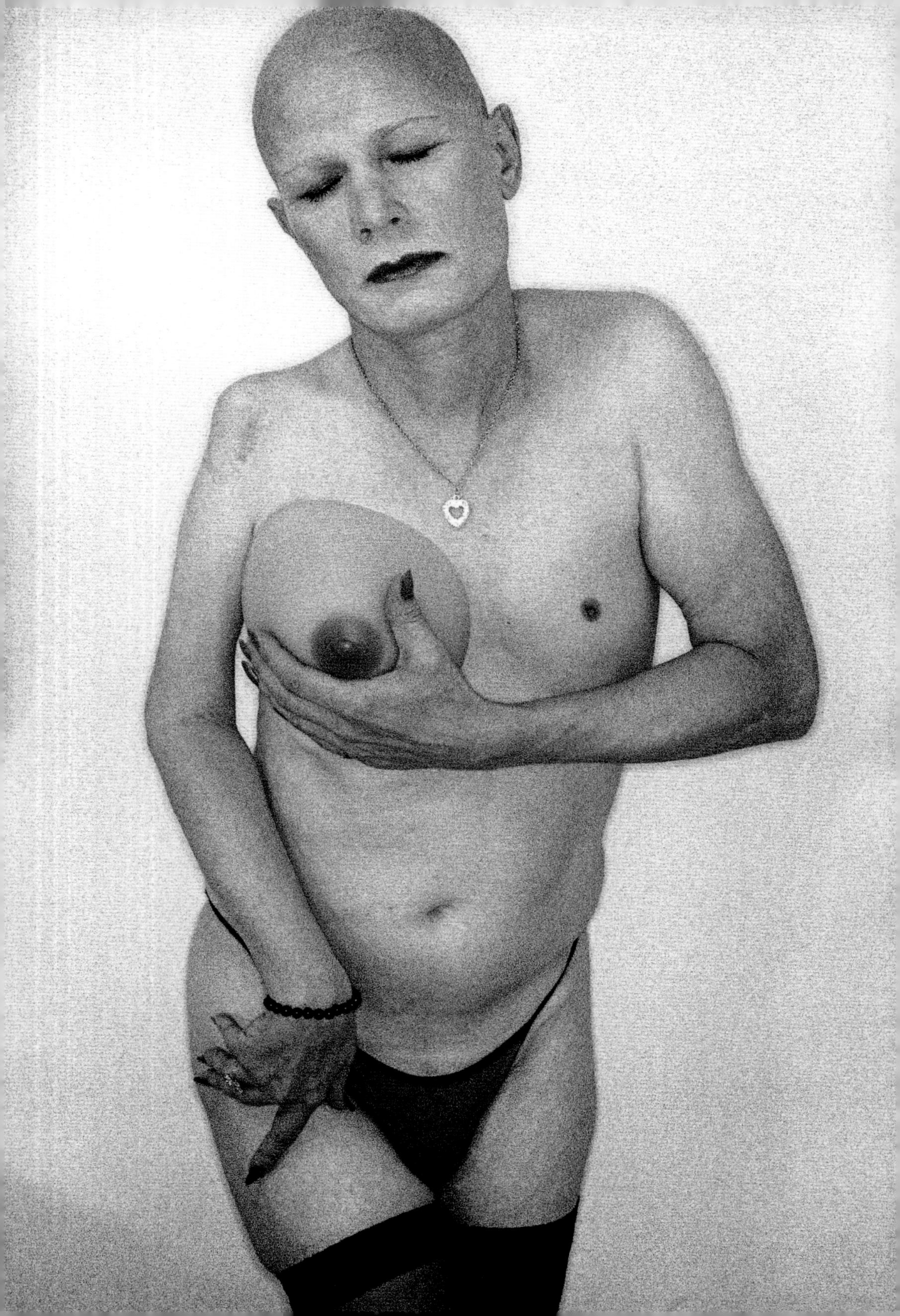

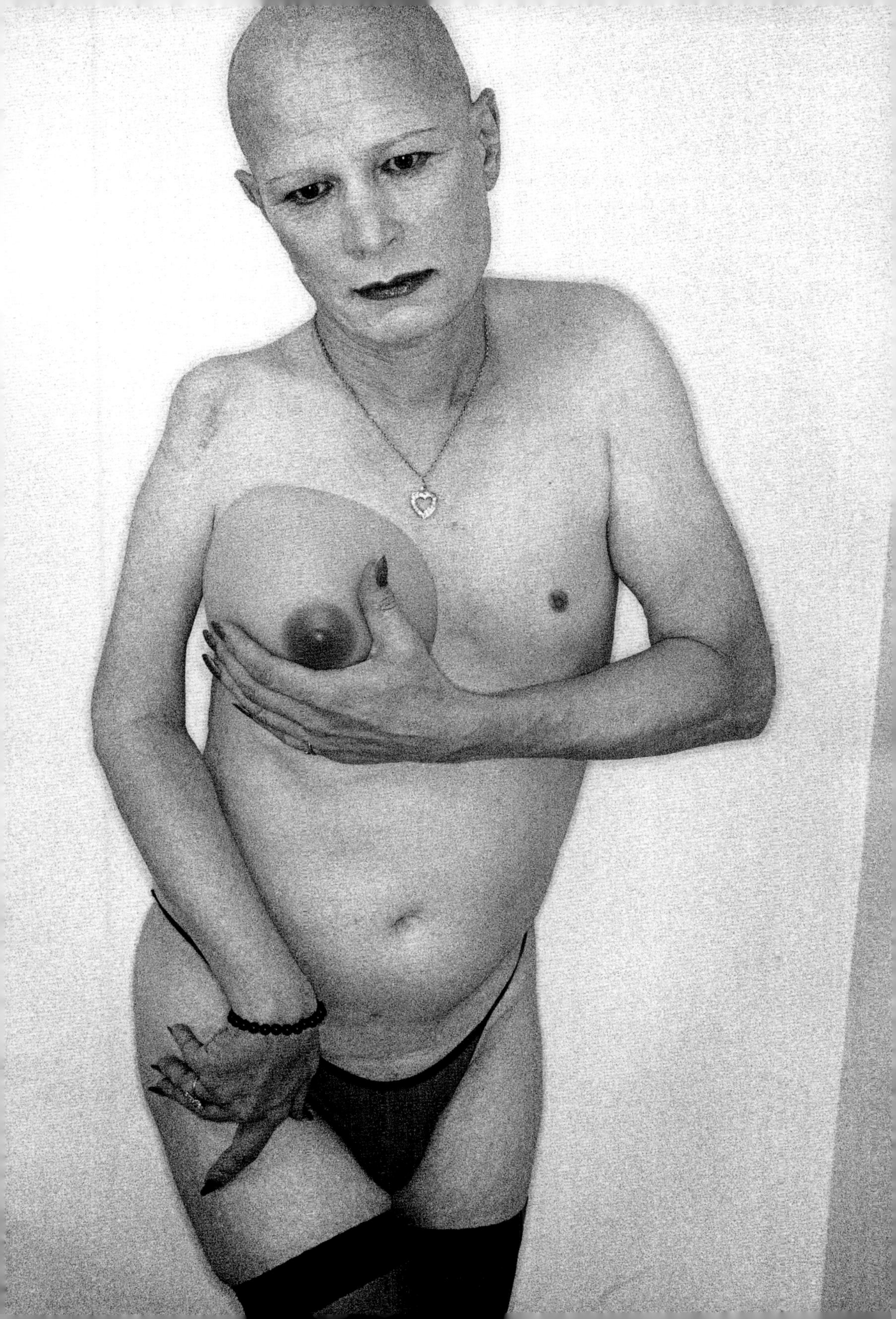

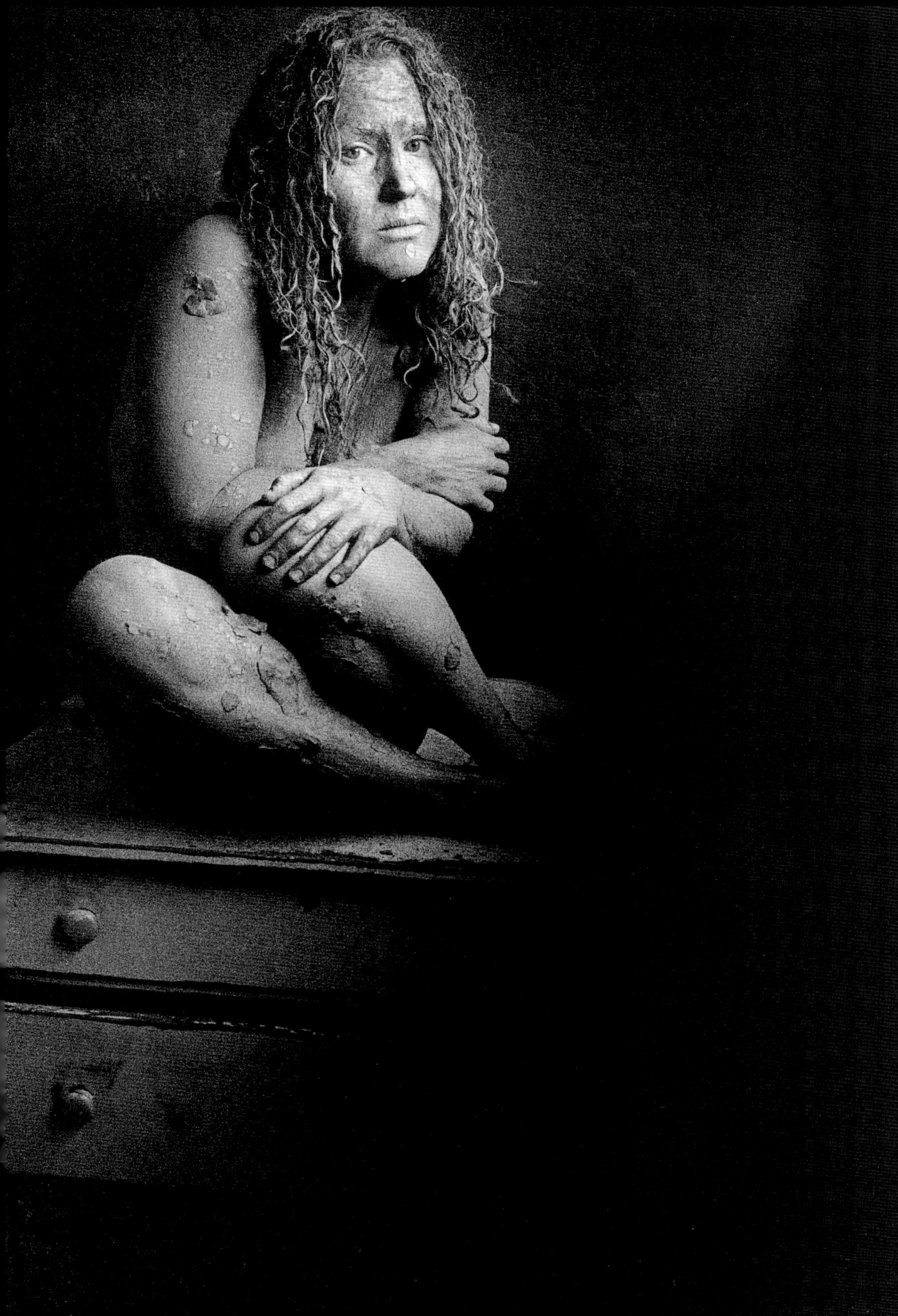

Renee

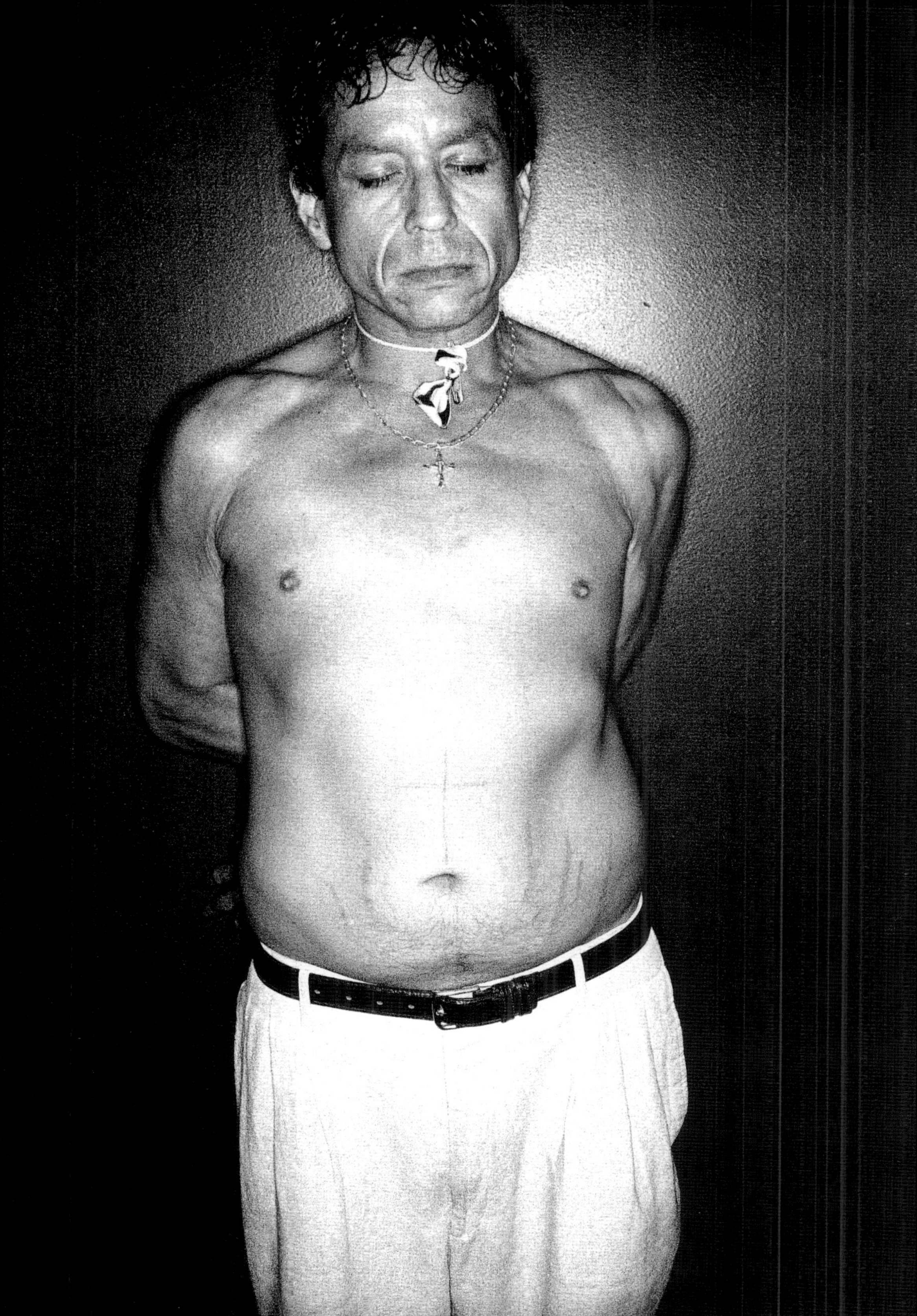

Robert

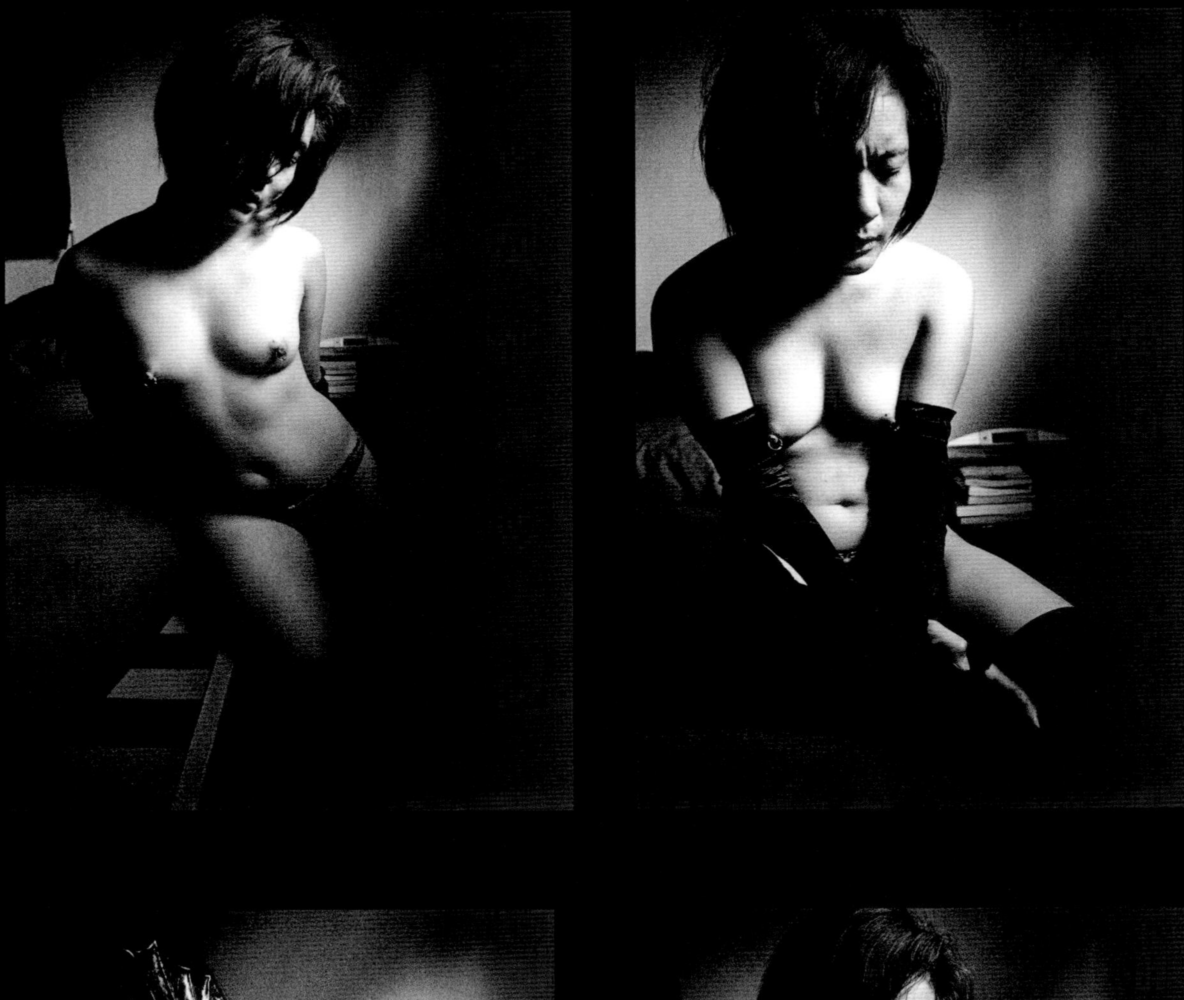

Kat 9

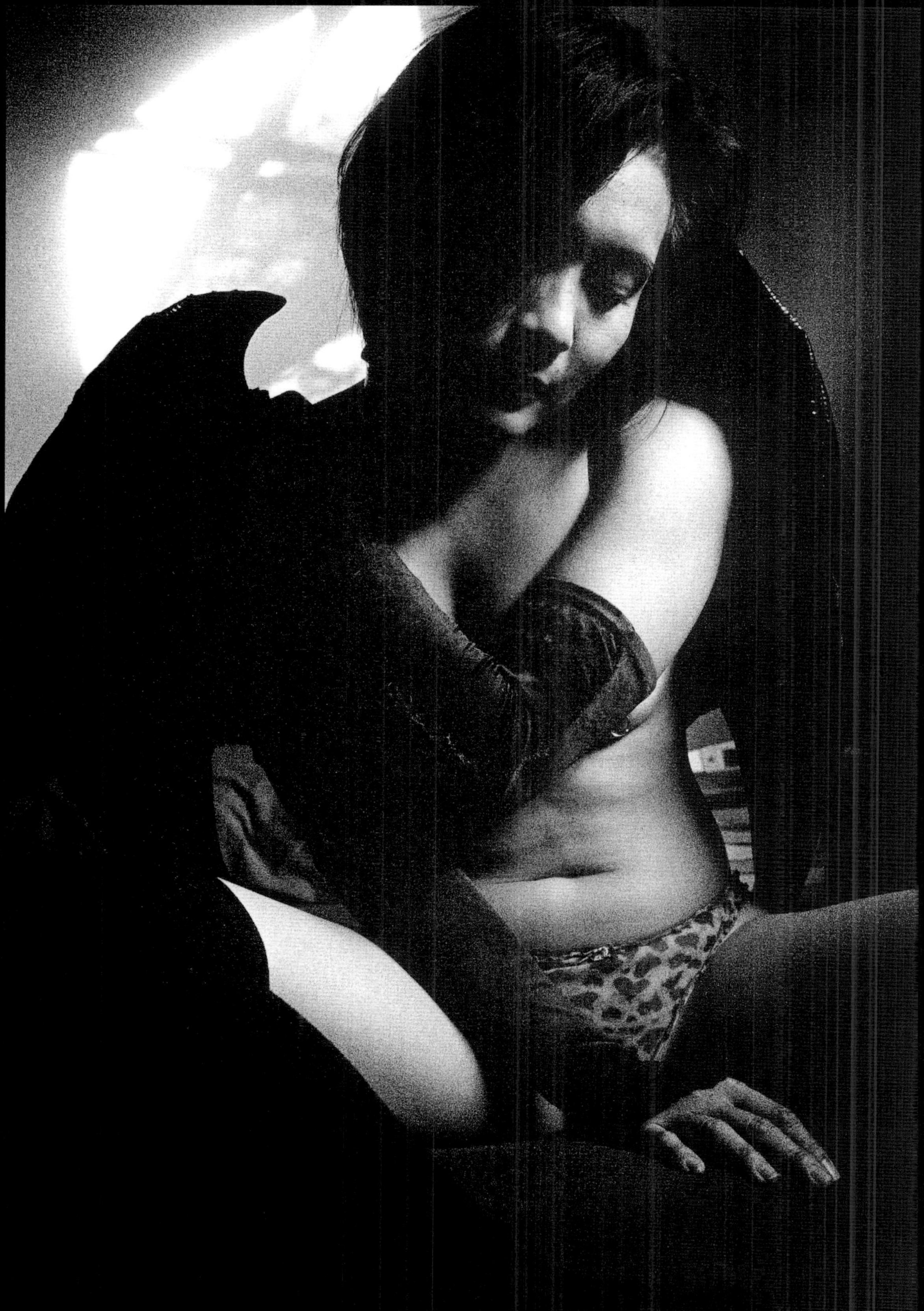

Kat 9

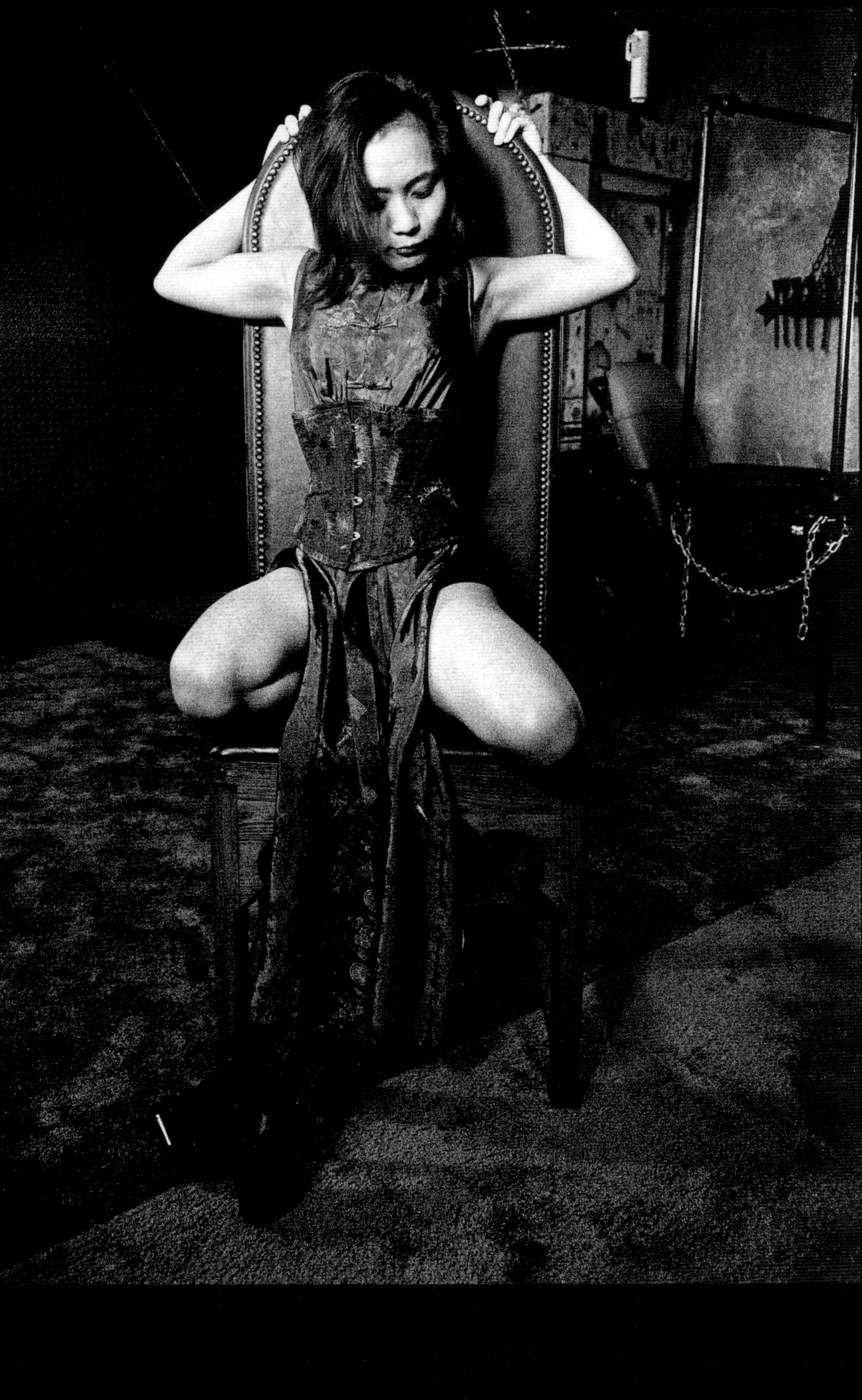

Kat 9

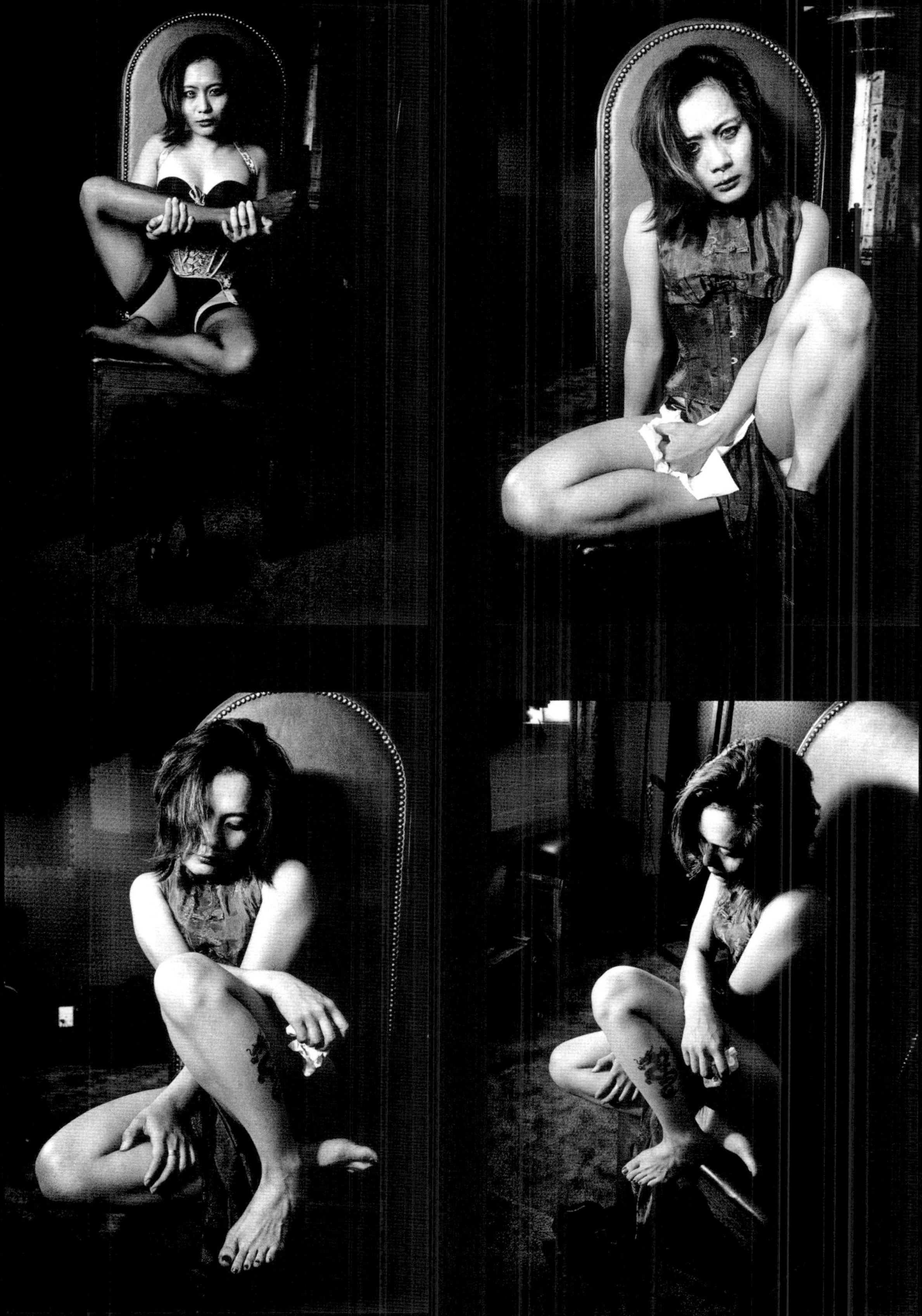

Kat 9

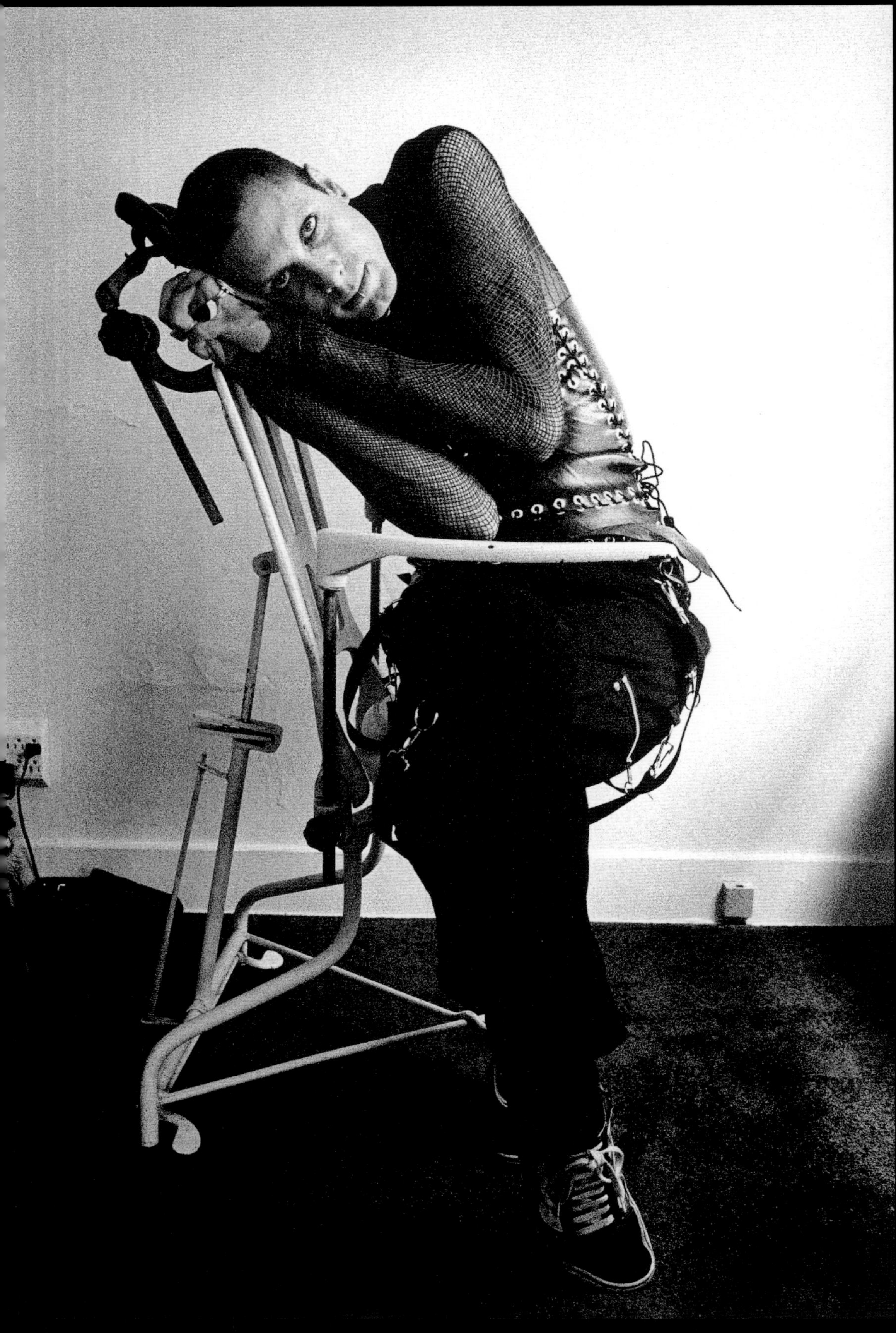

Reverend Death

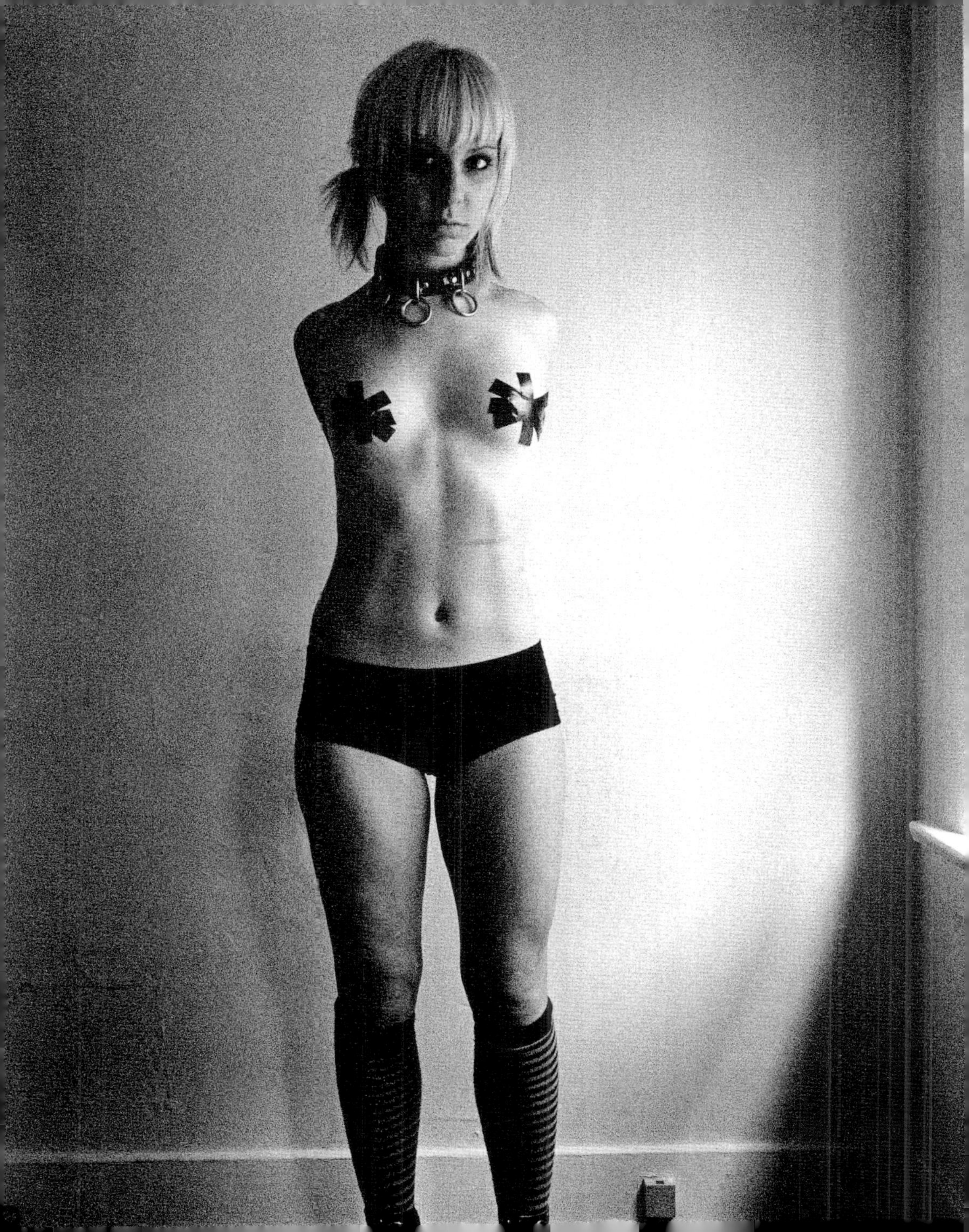

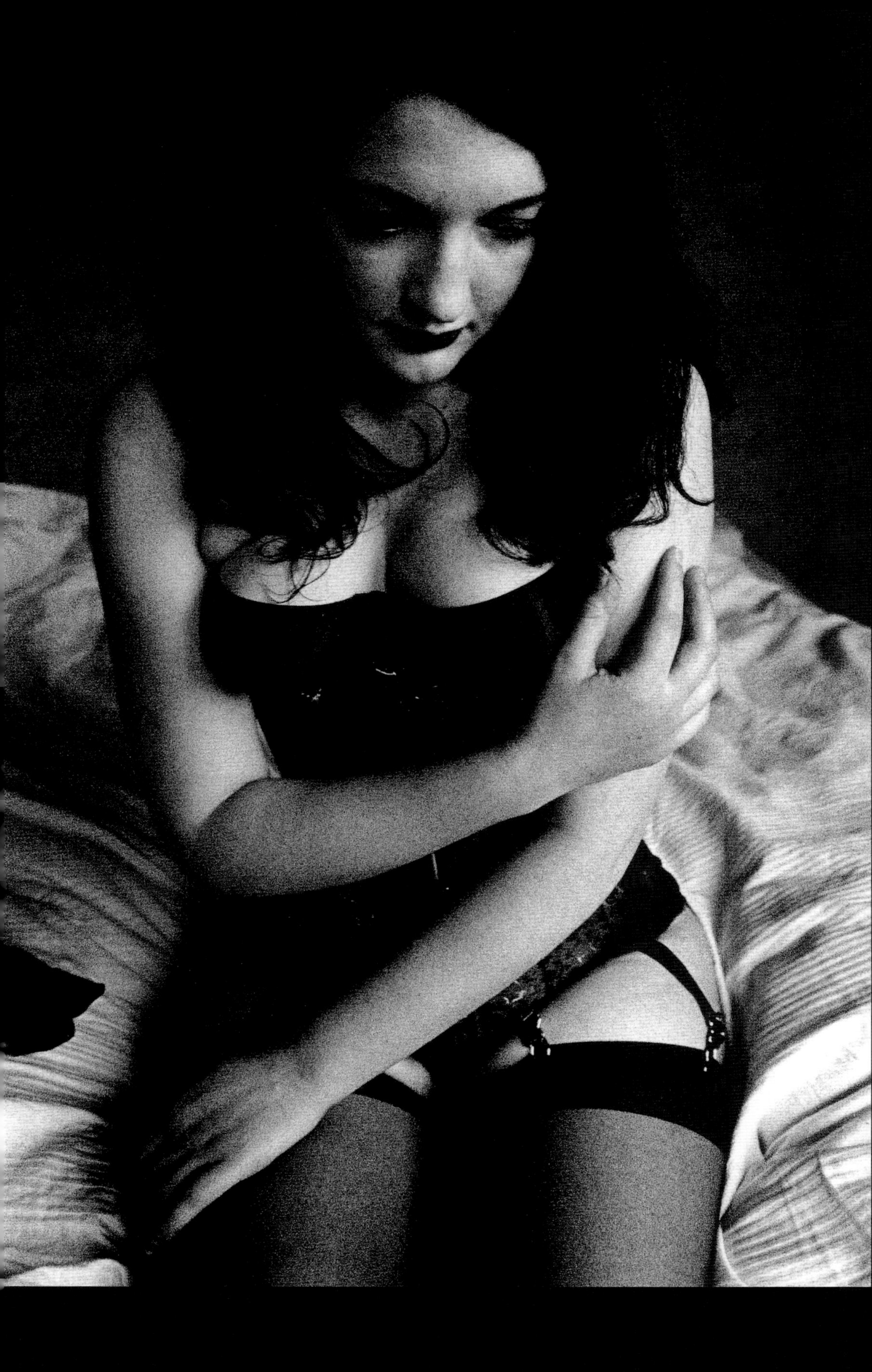

Virginia

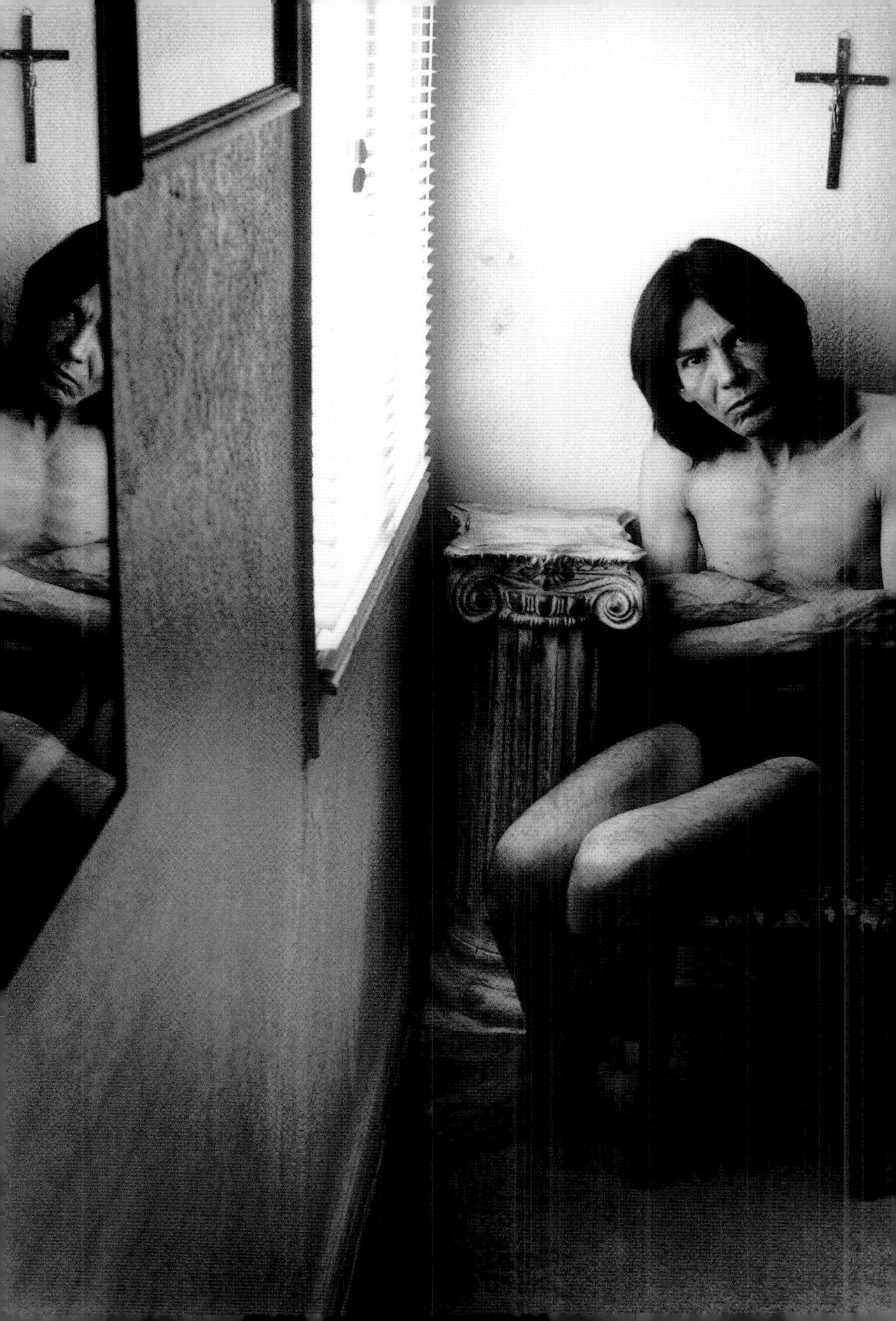

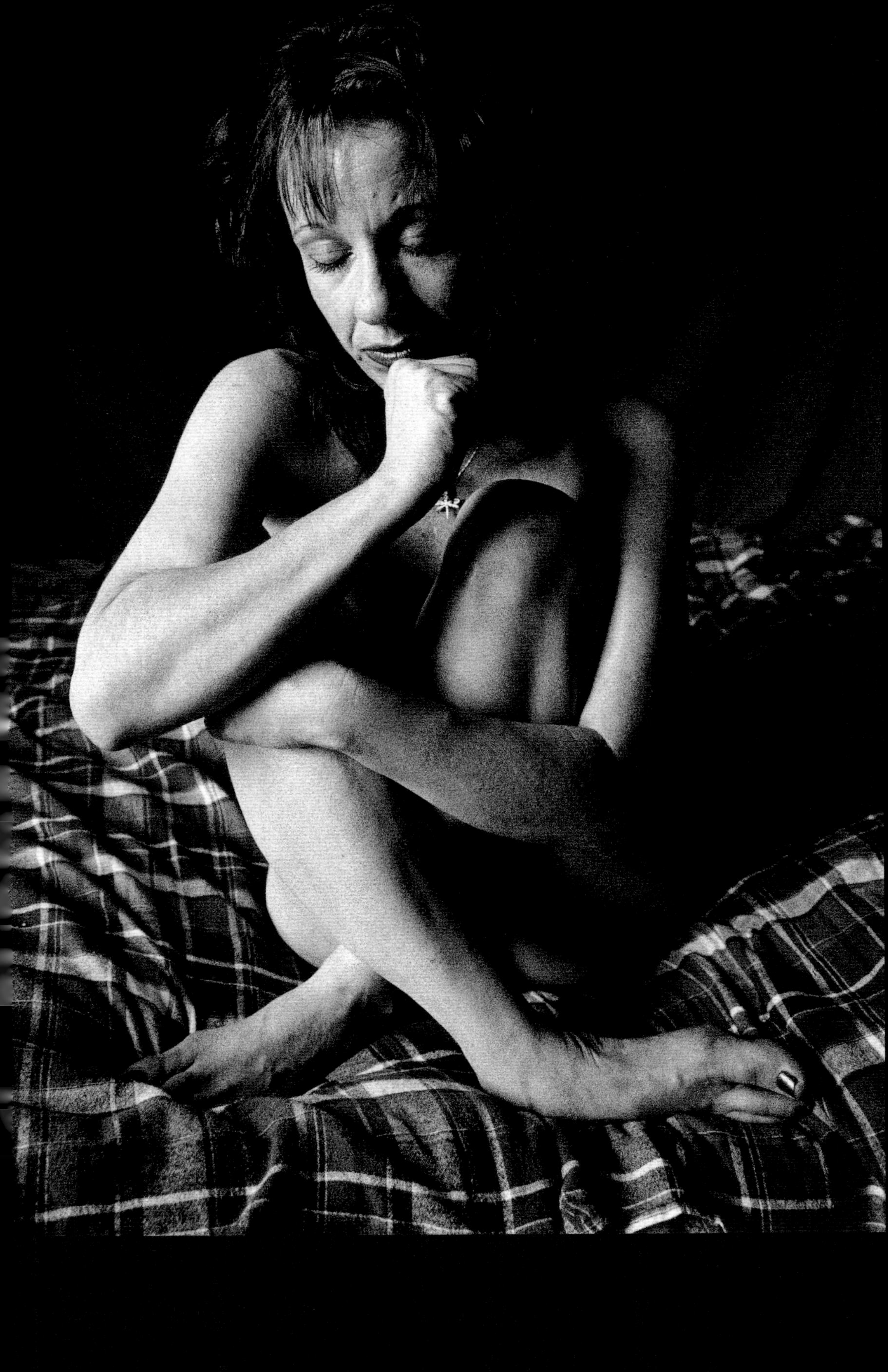

Tazma

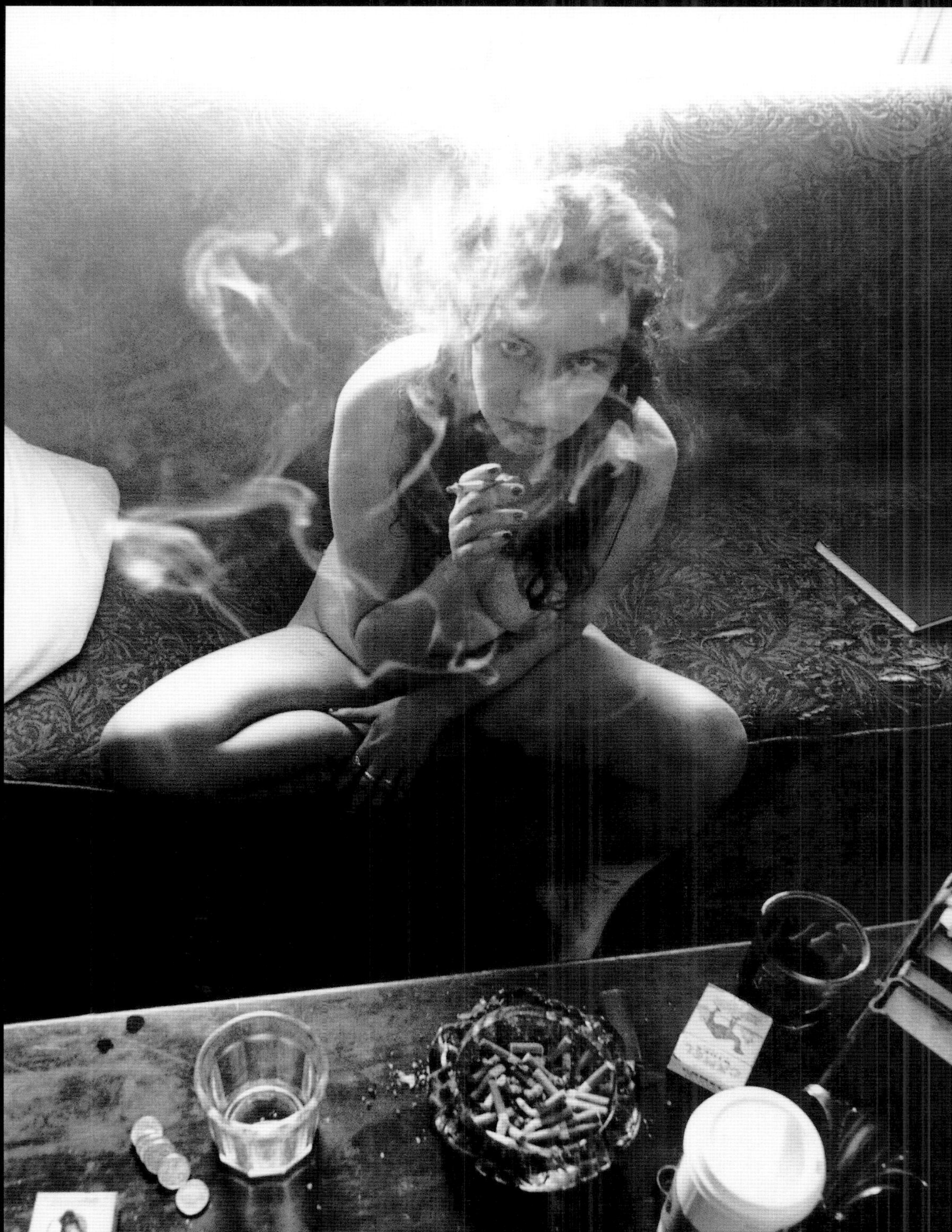

Spanky

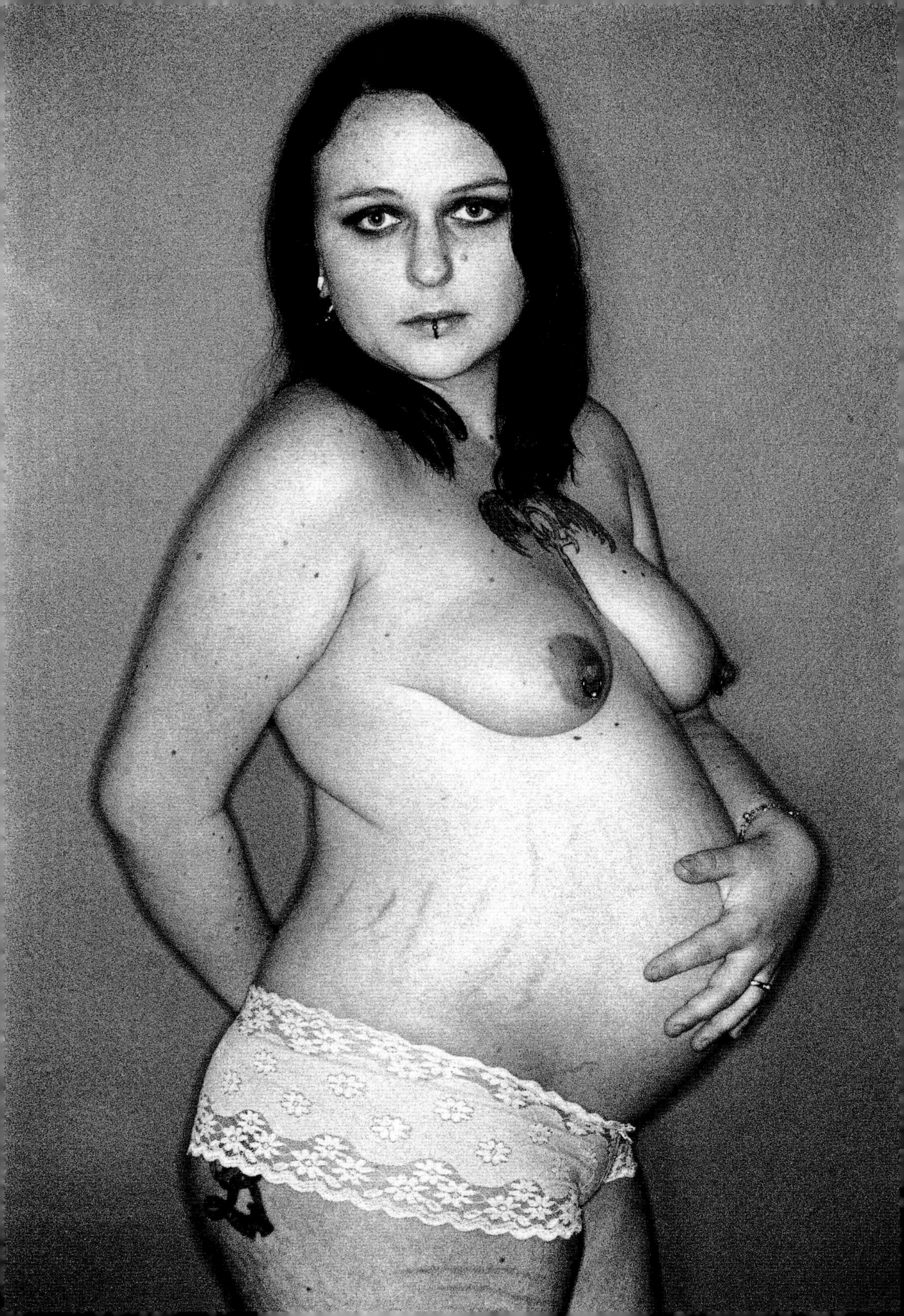

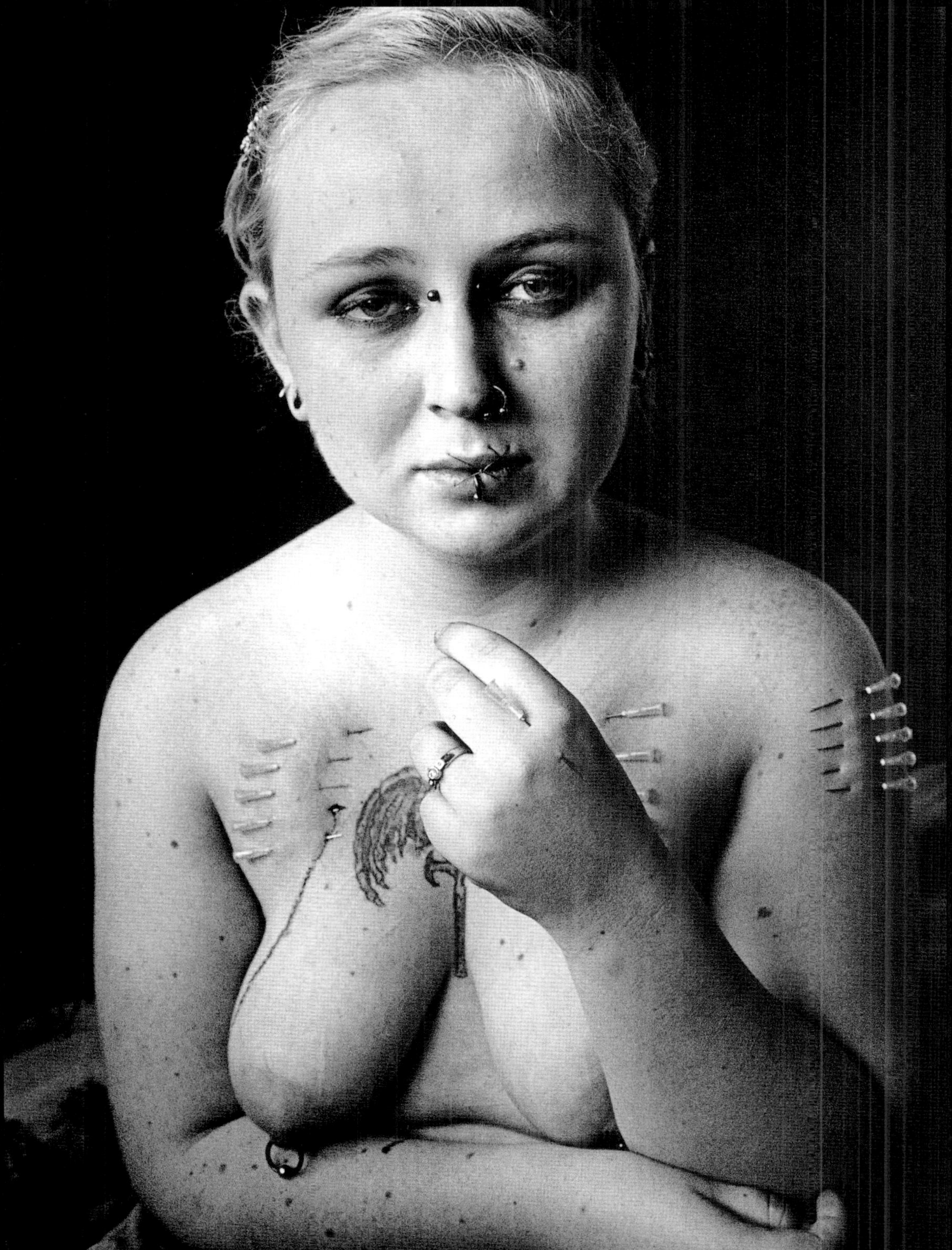

Little Bit

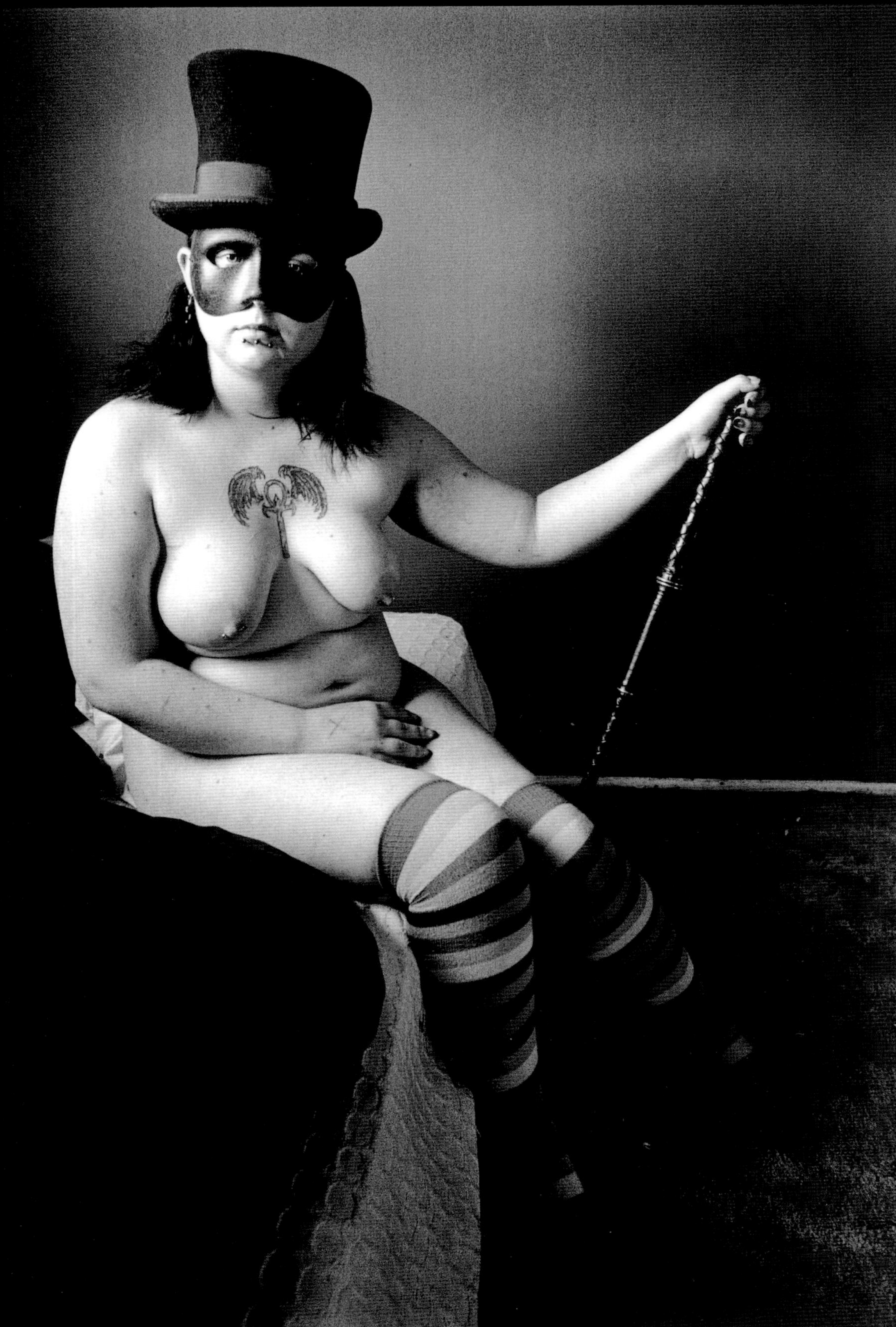

Little Bit

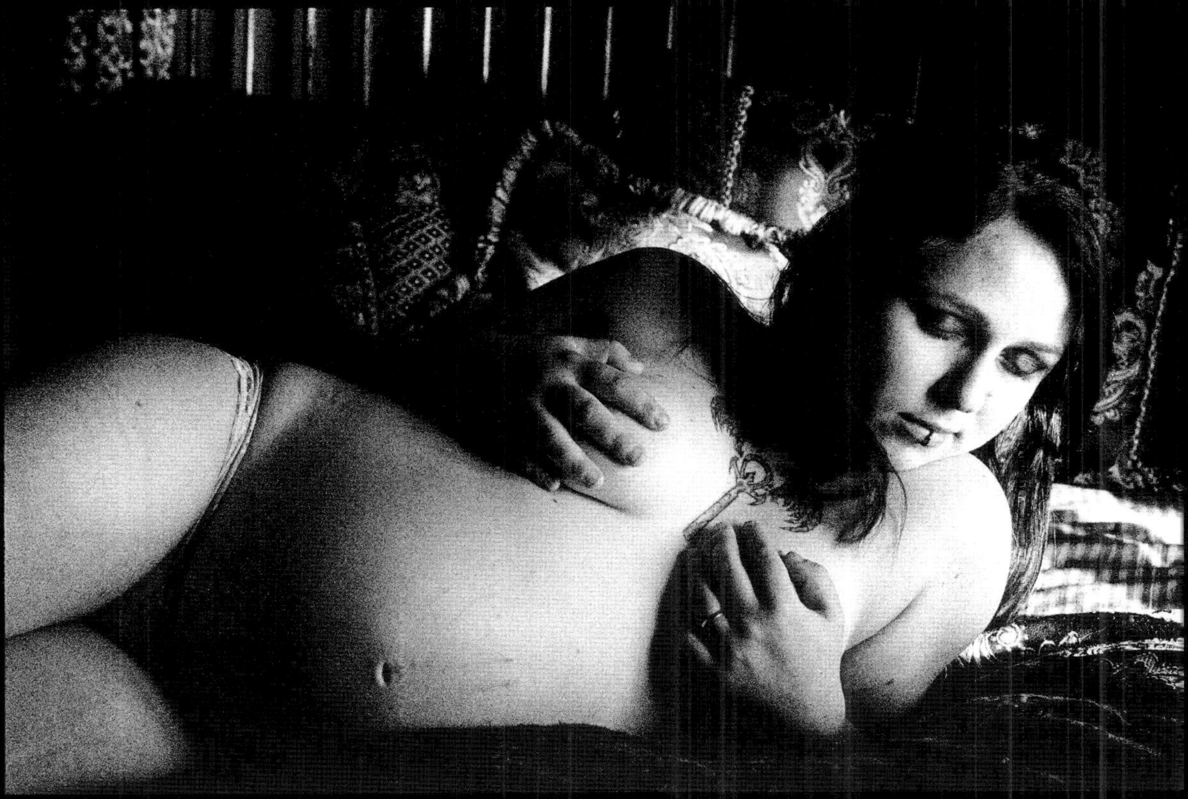

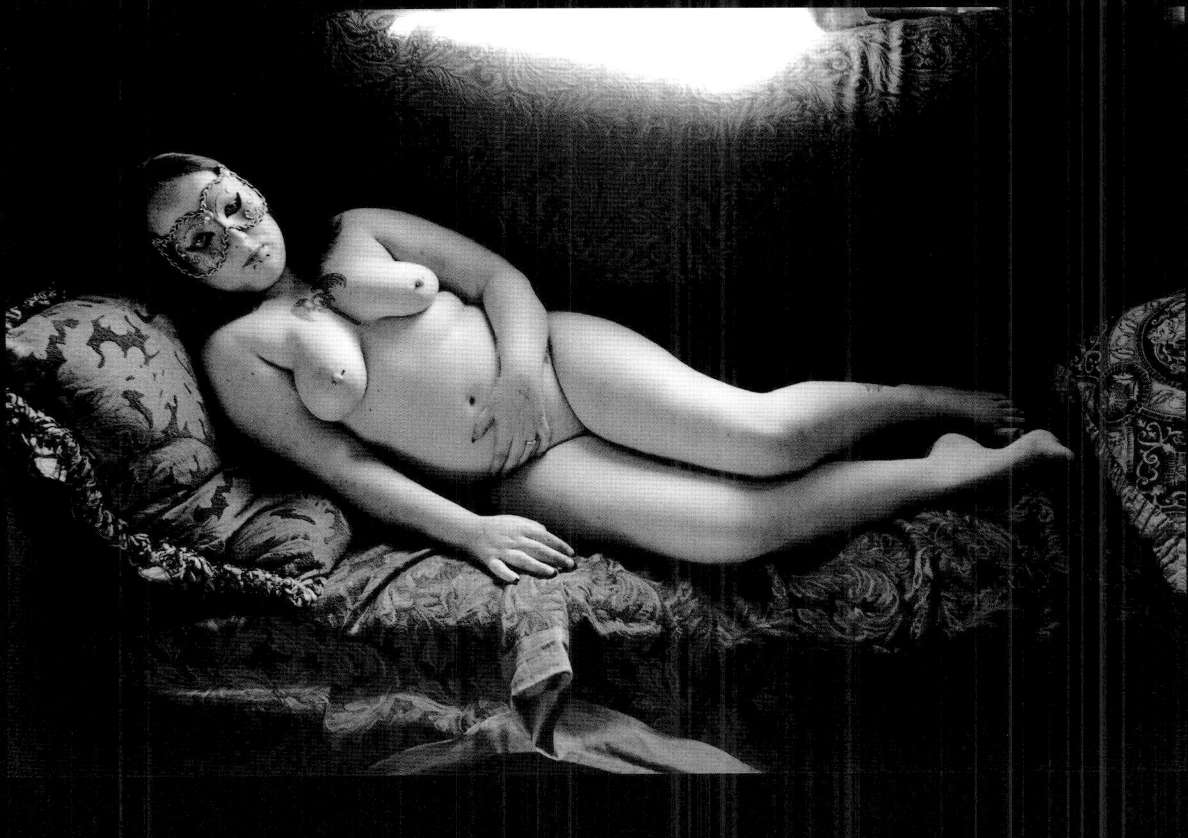

Little Bit

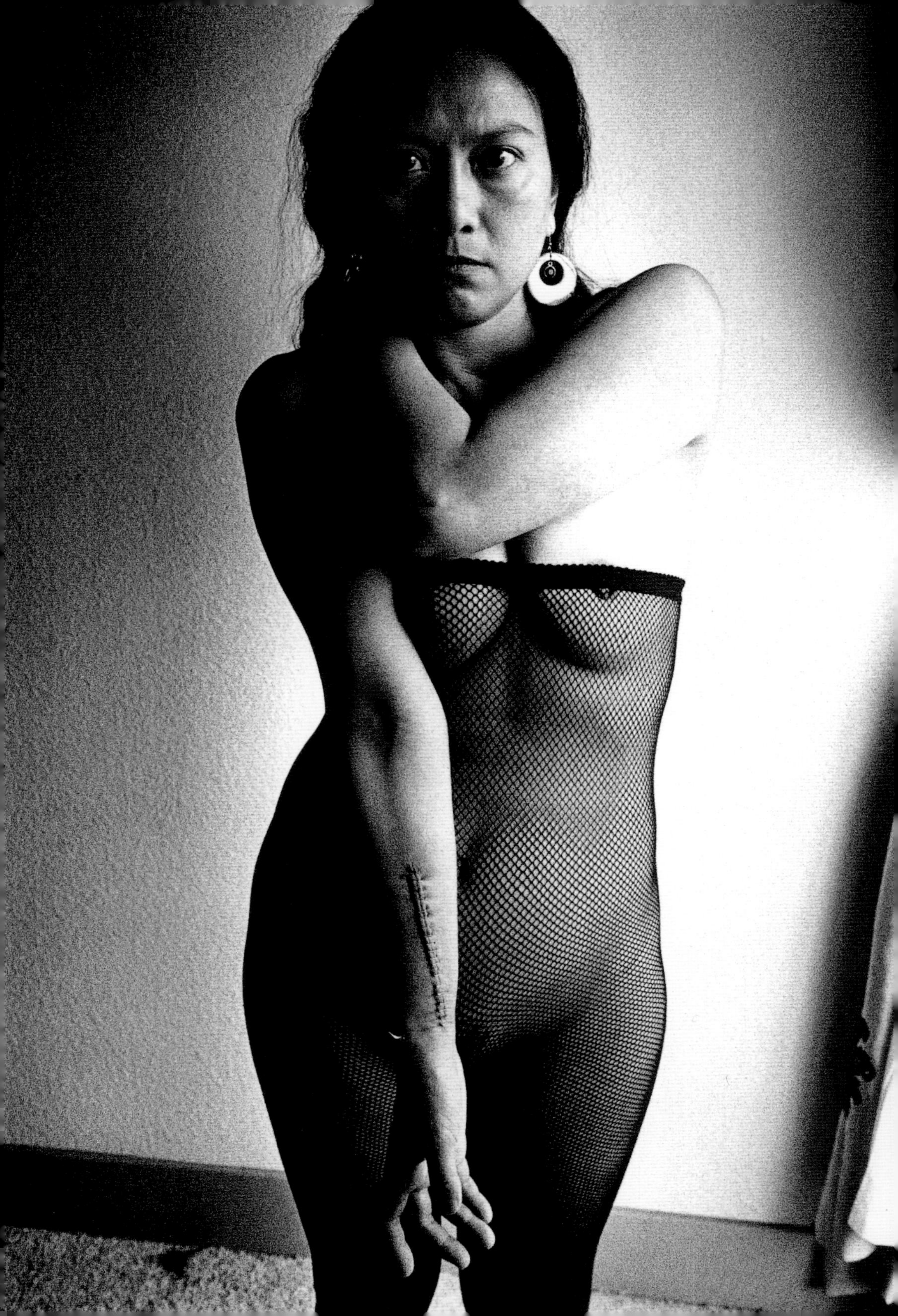

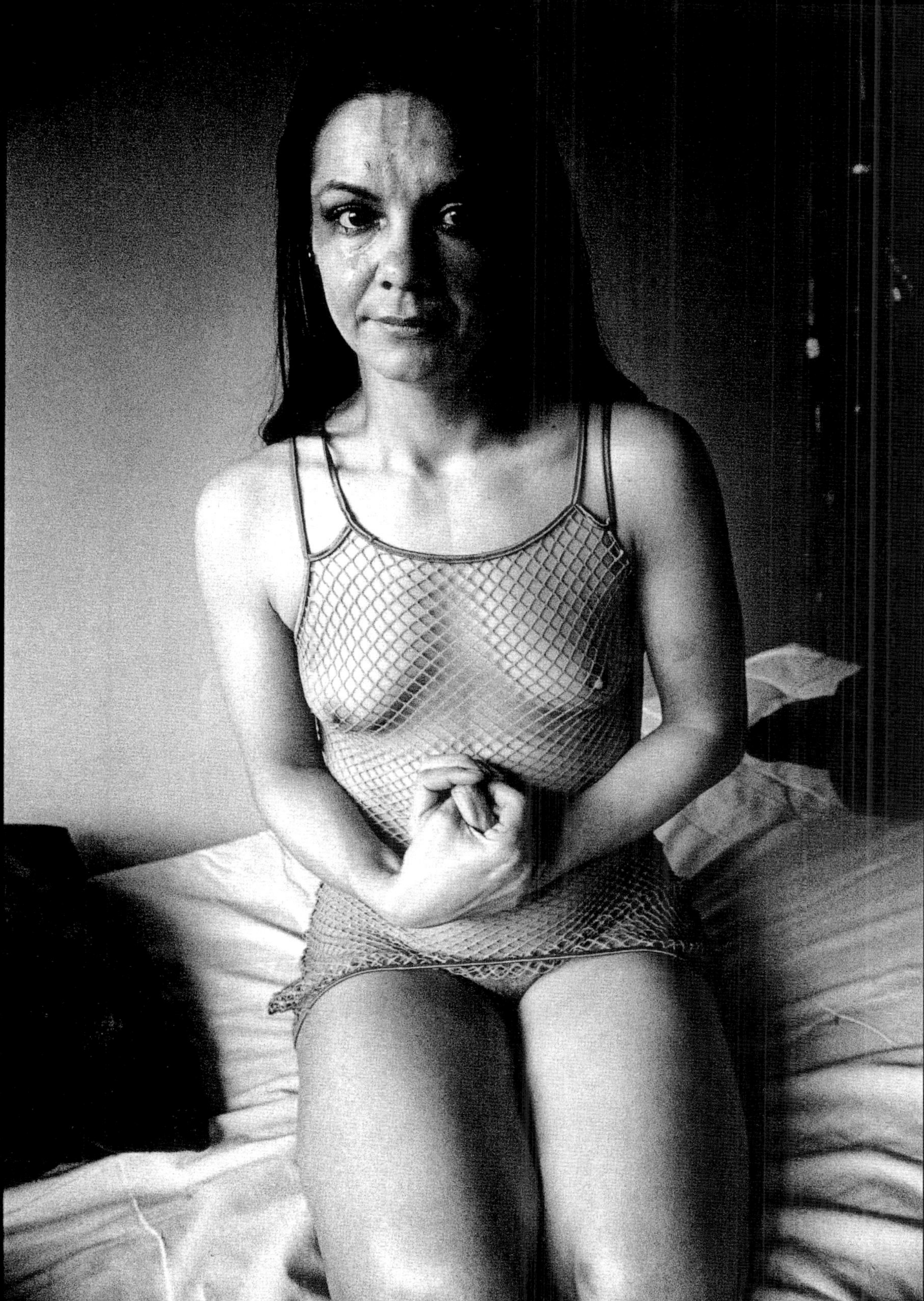

Luna

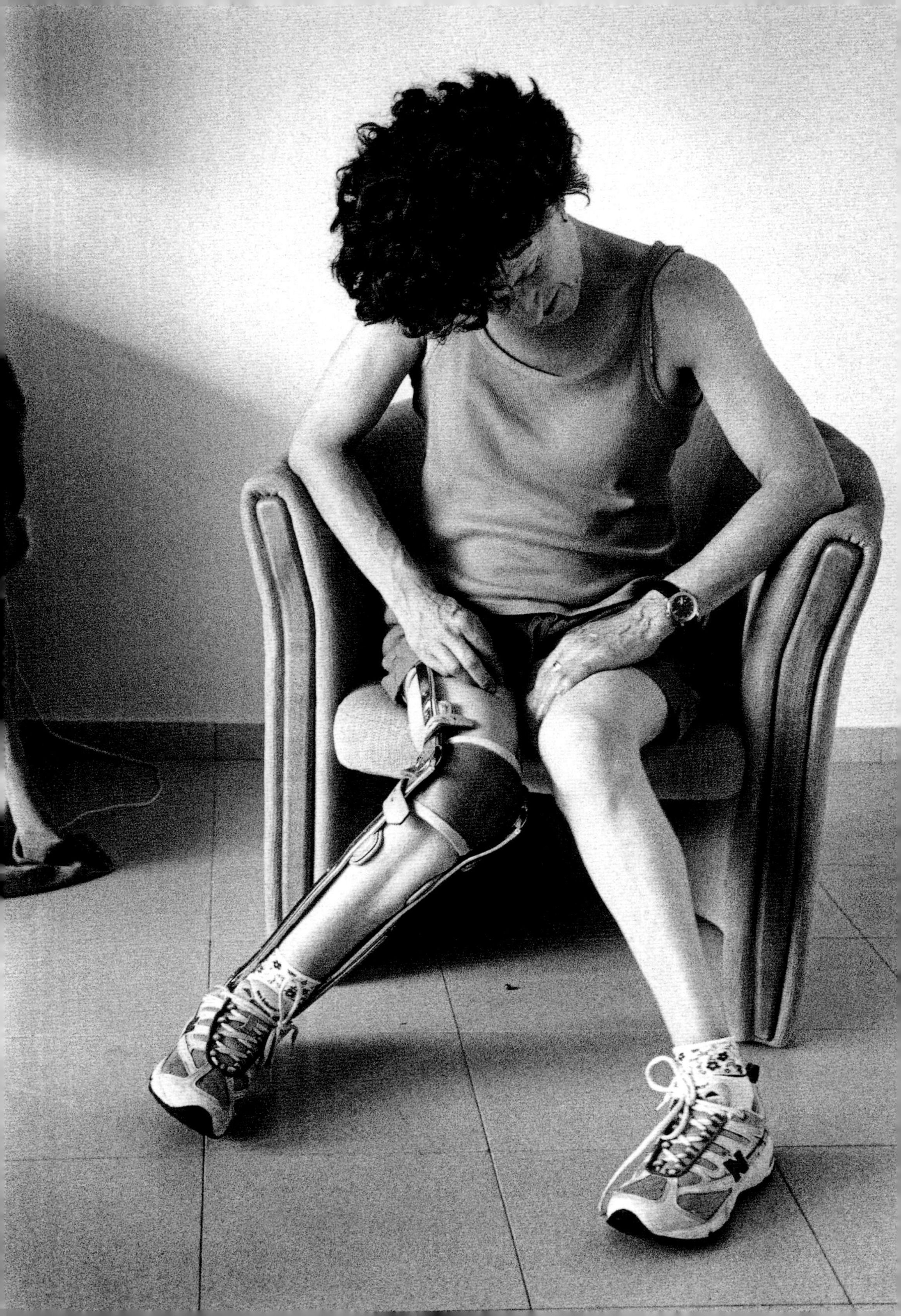

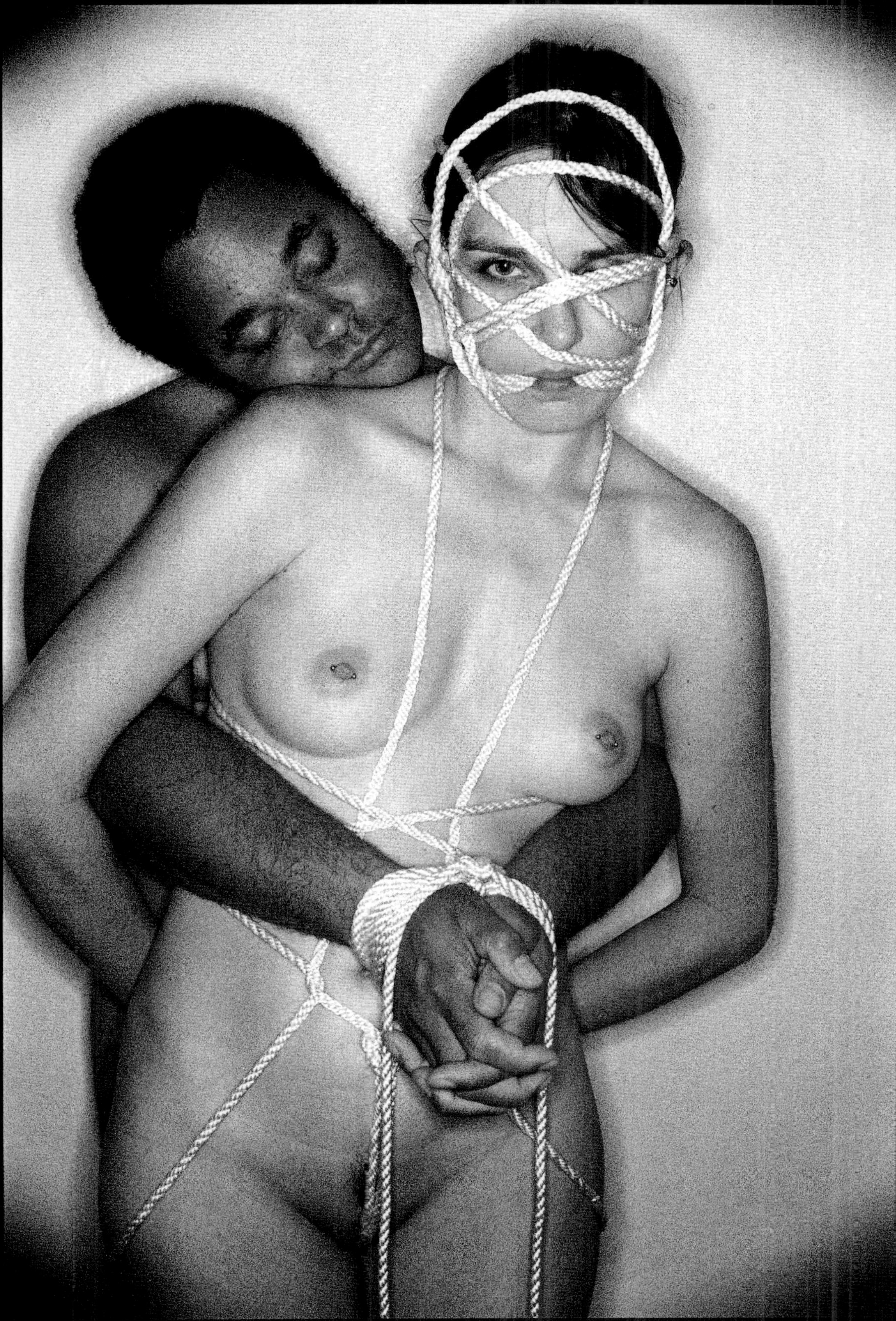

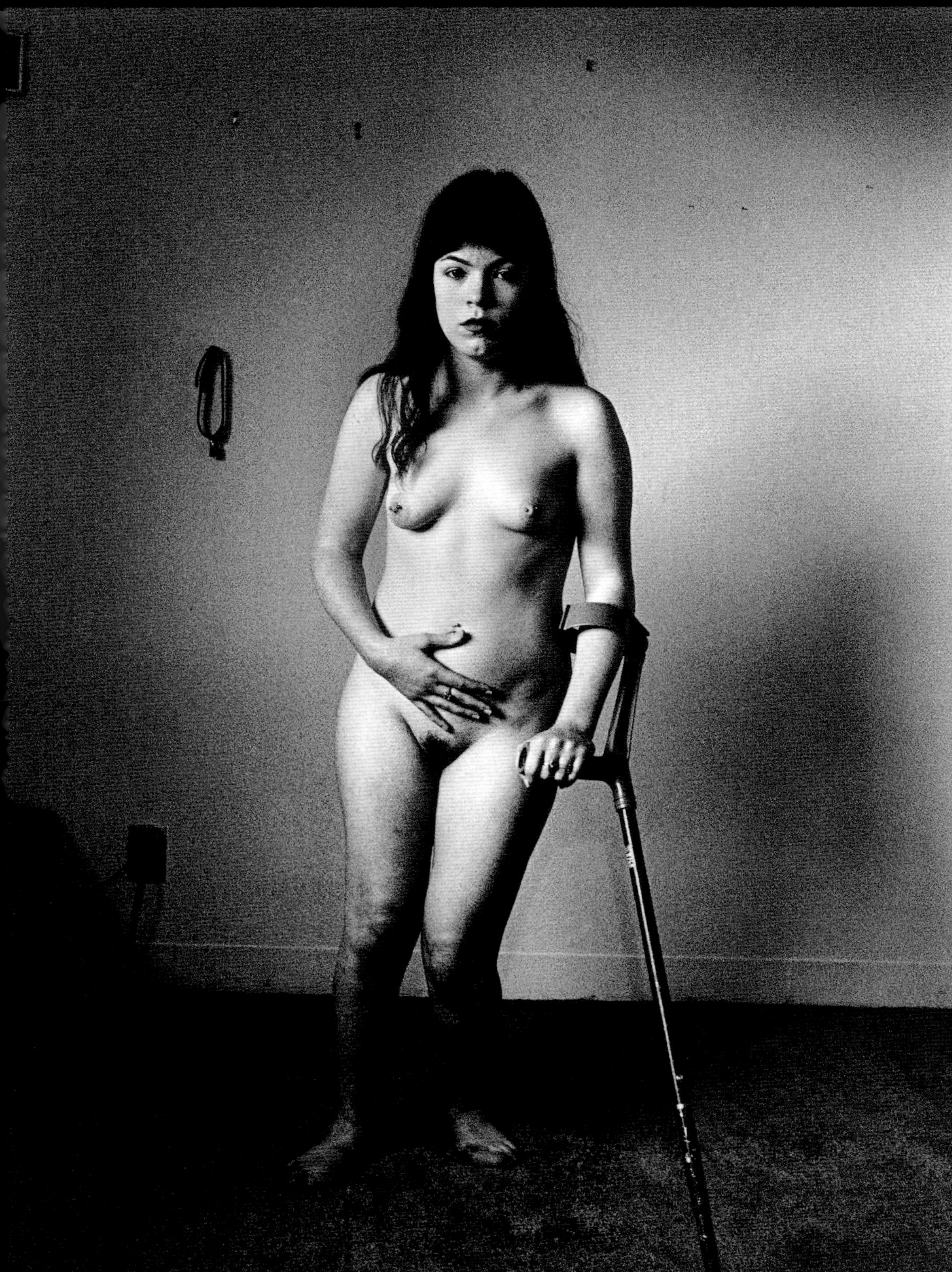

Shelly

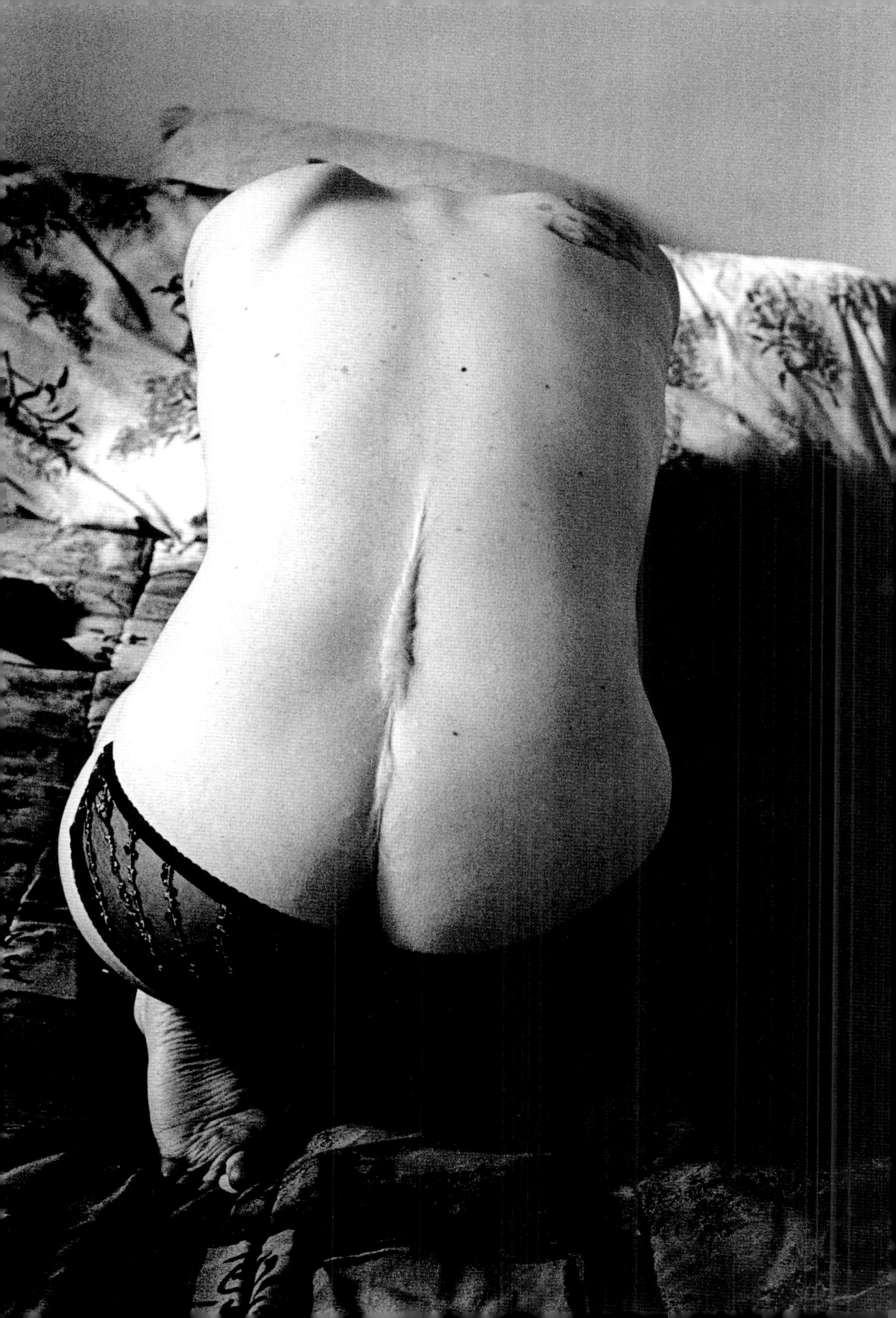

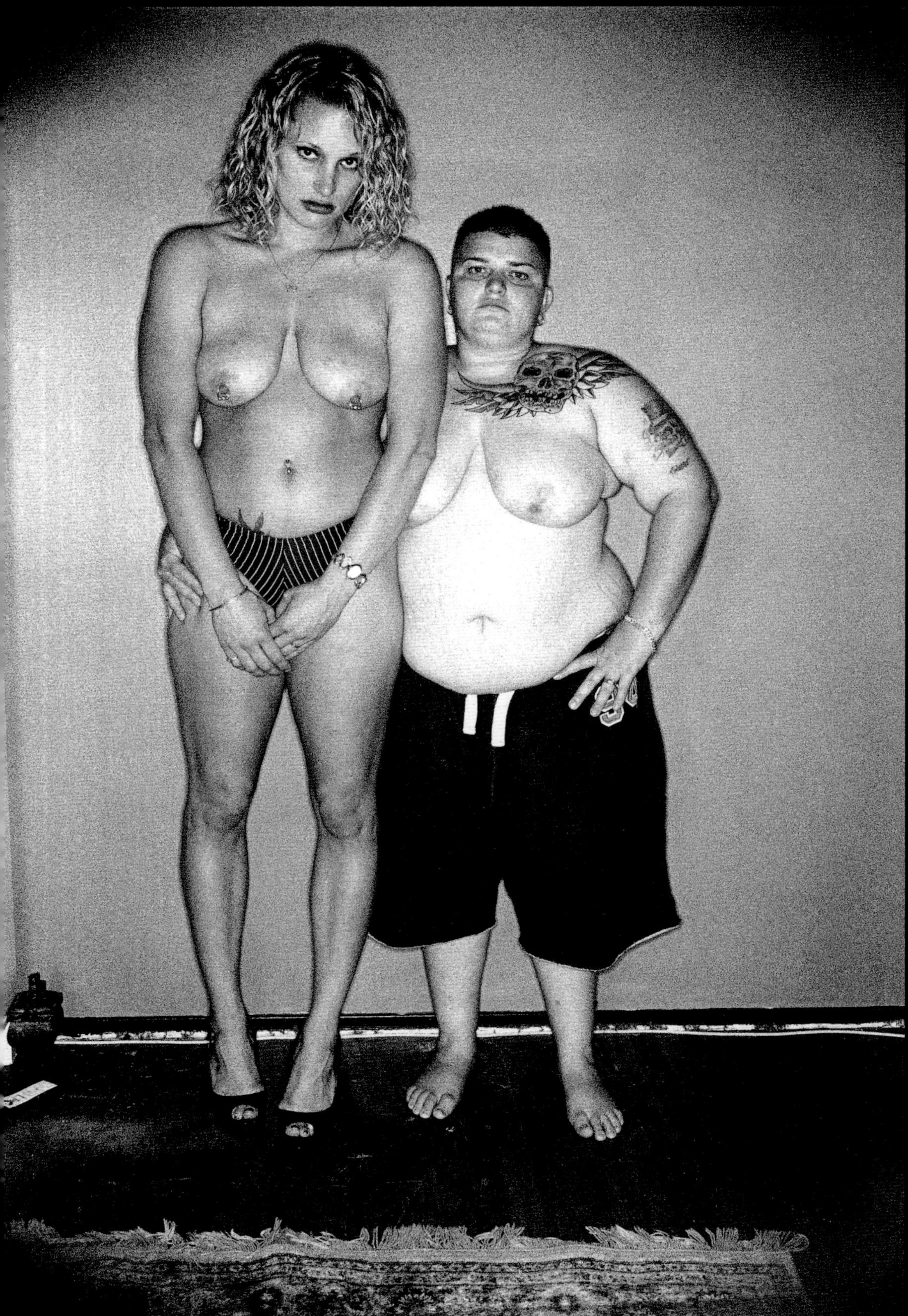

Candace & Dez

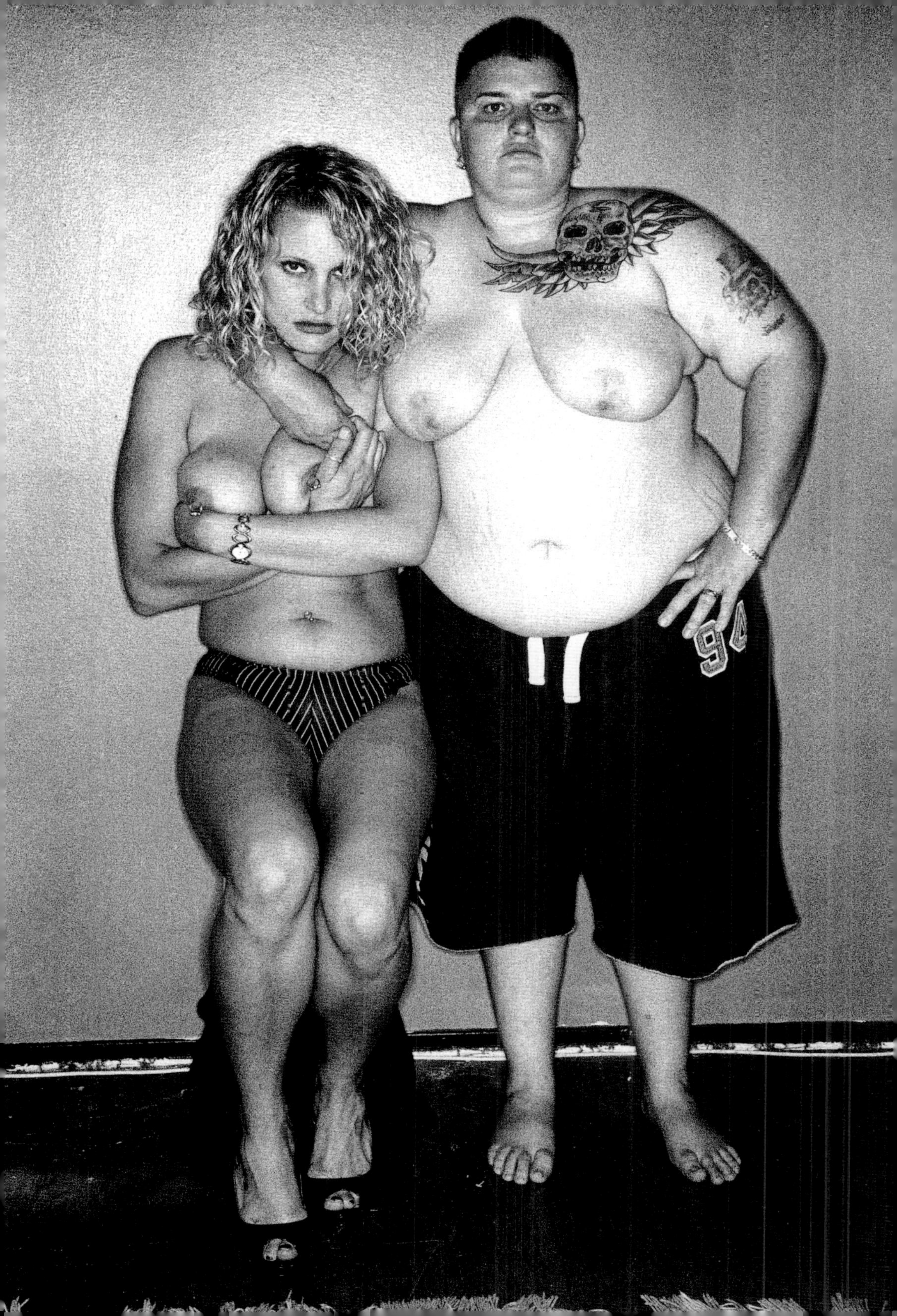

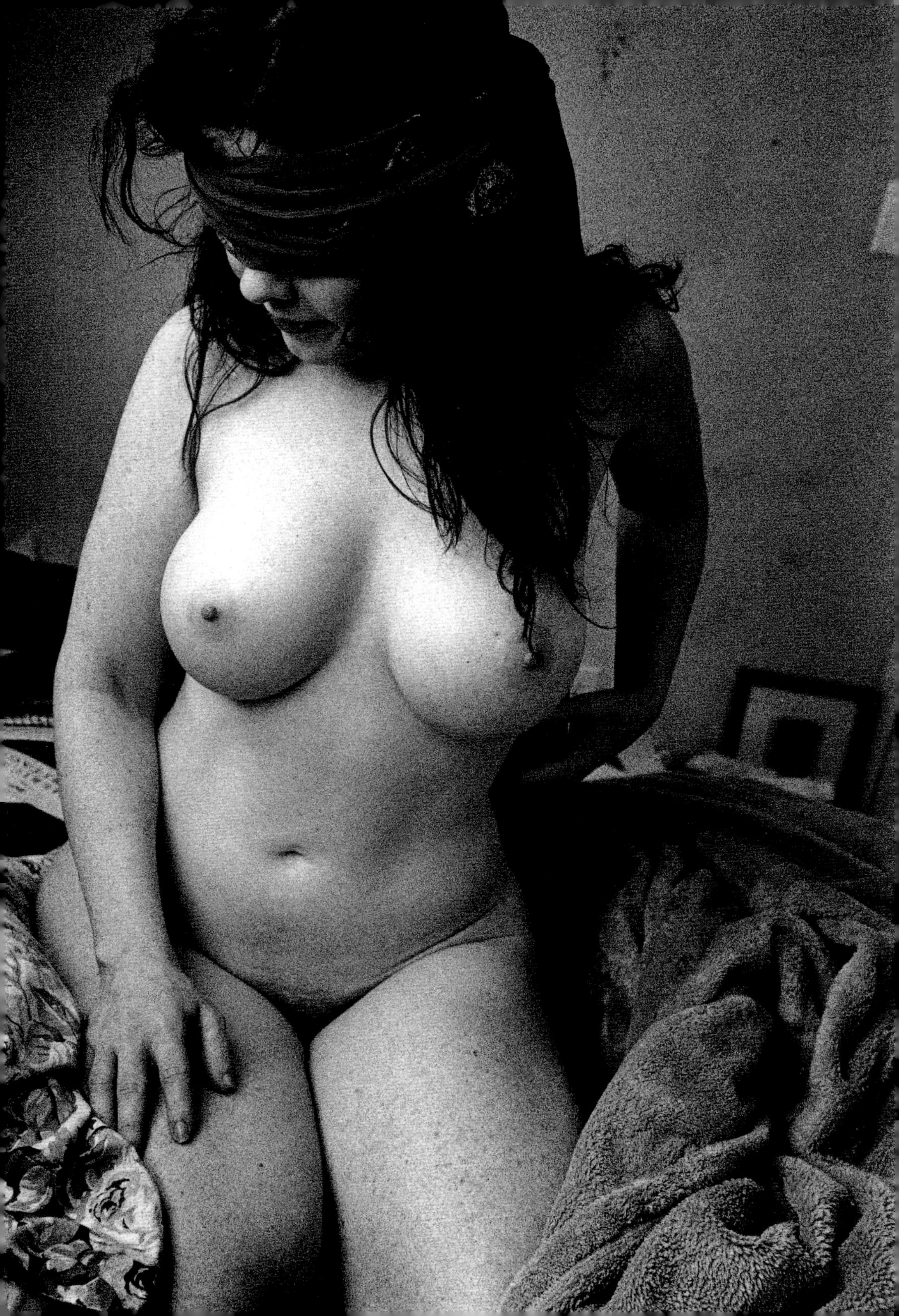

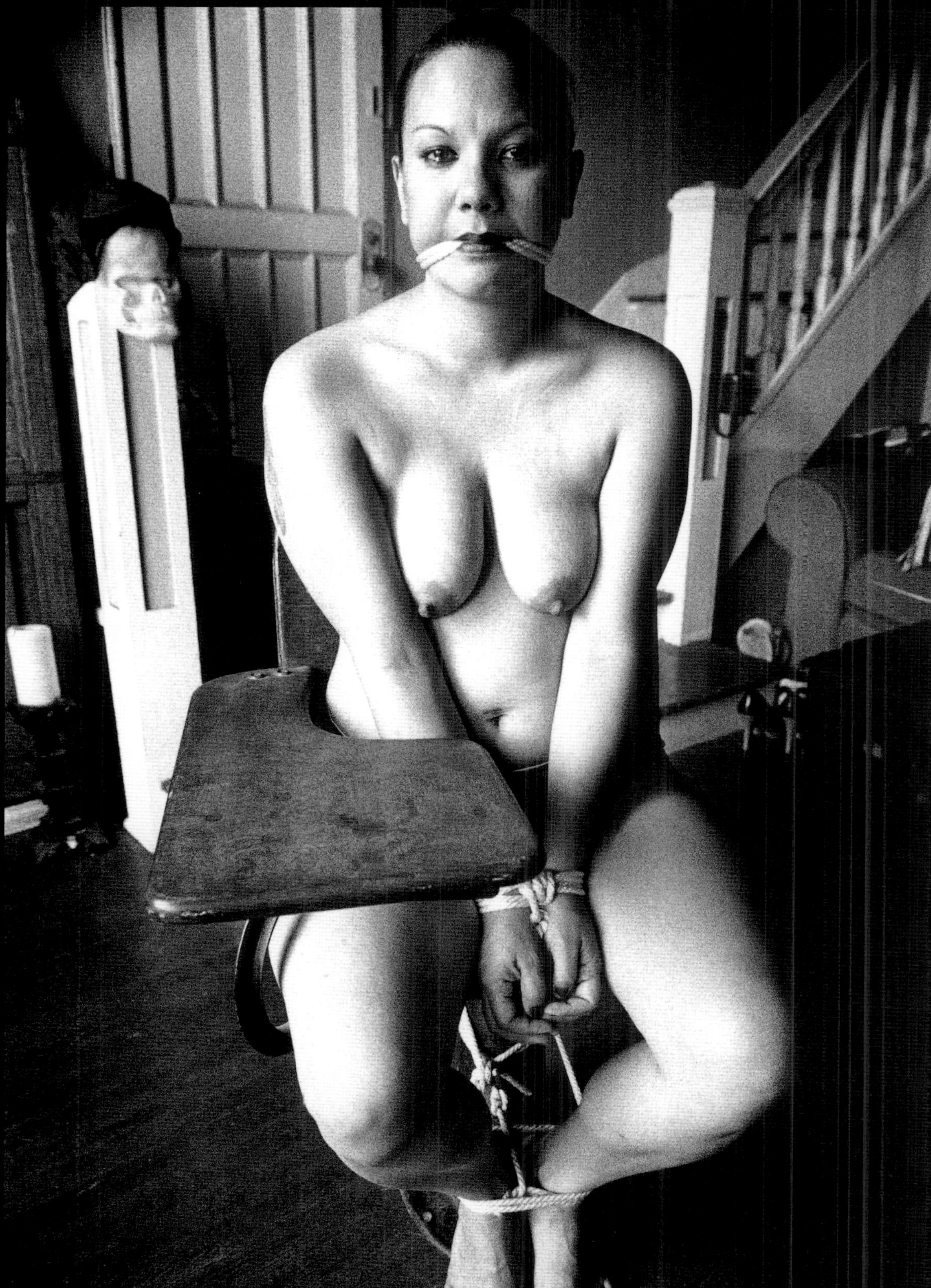

Michelle

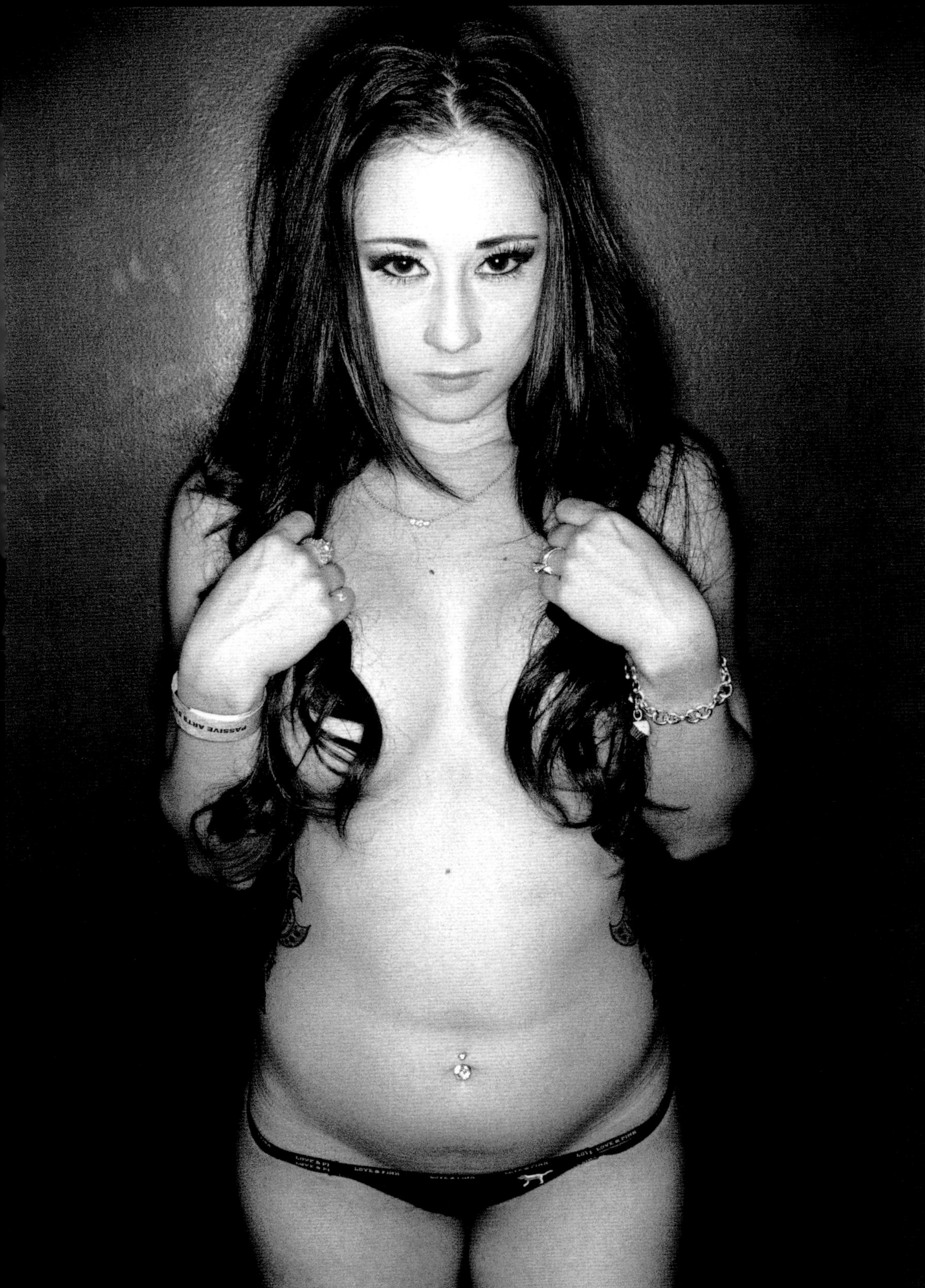

Schwinn

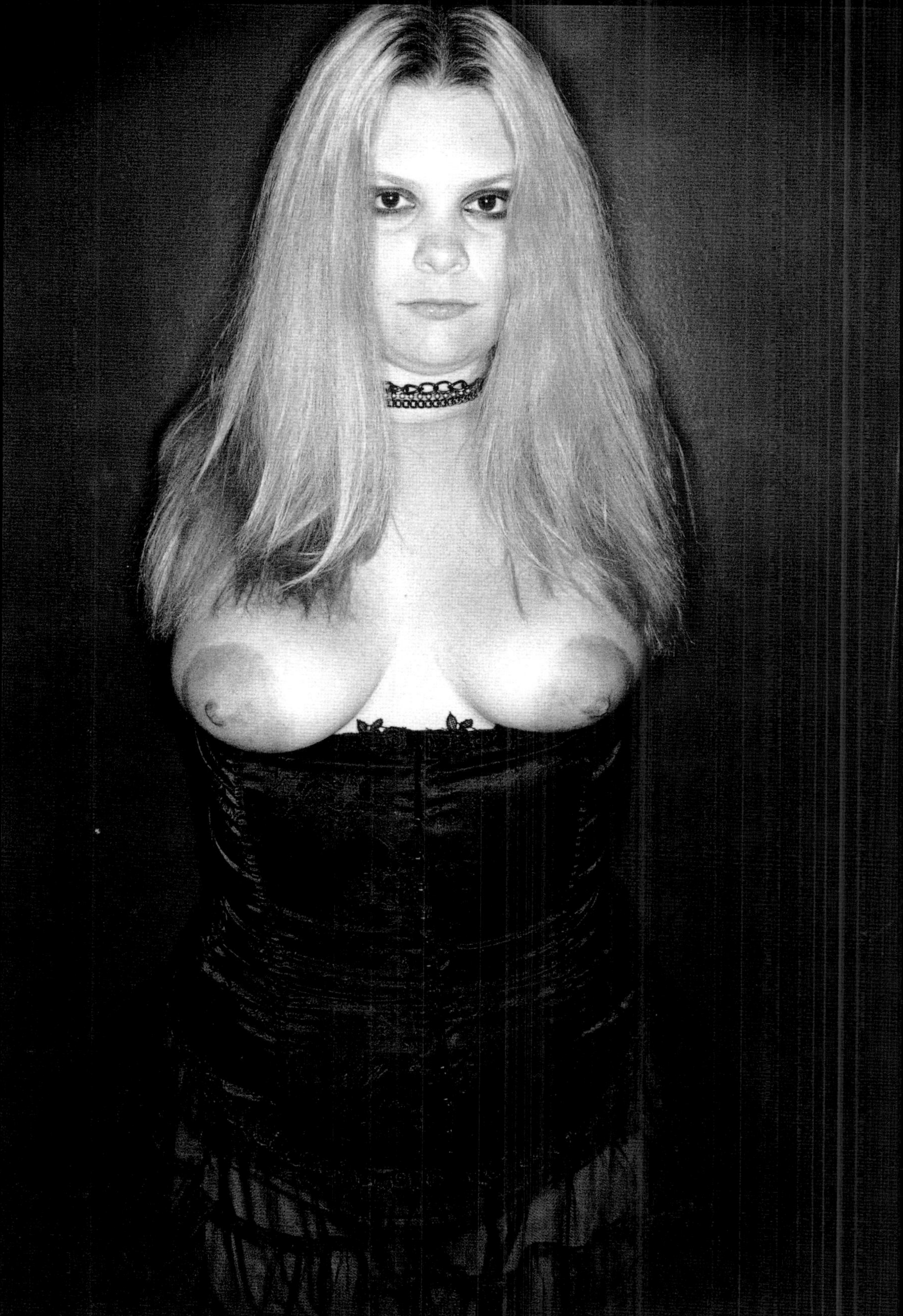

Shy

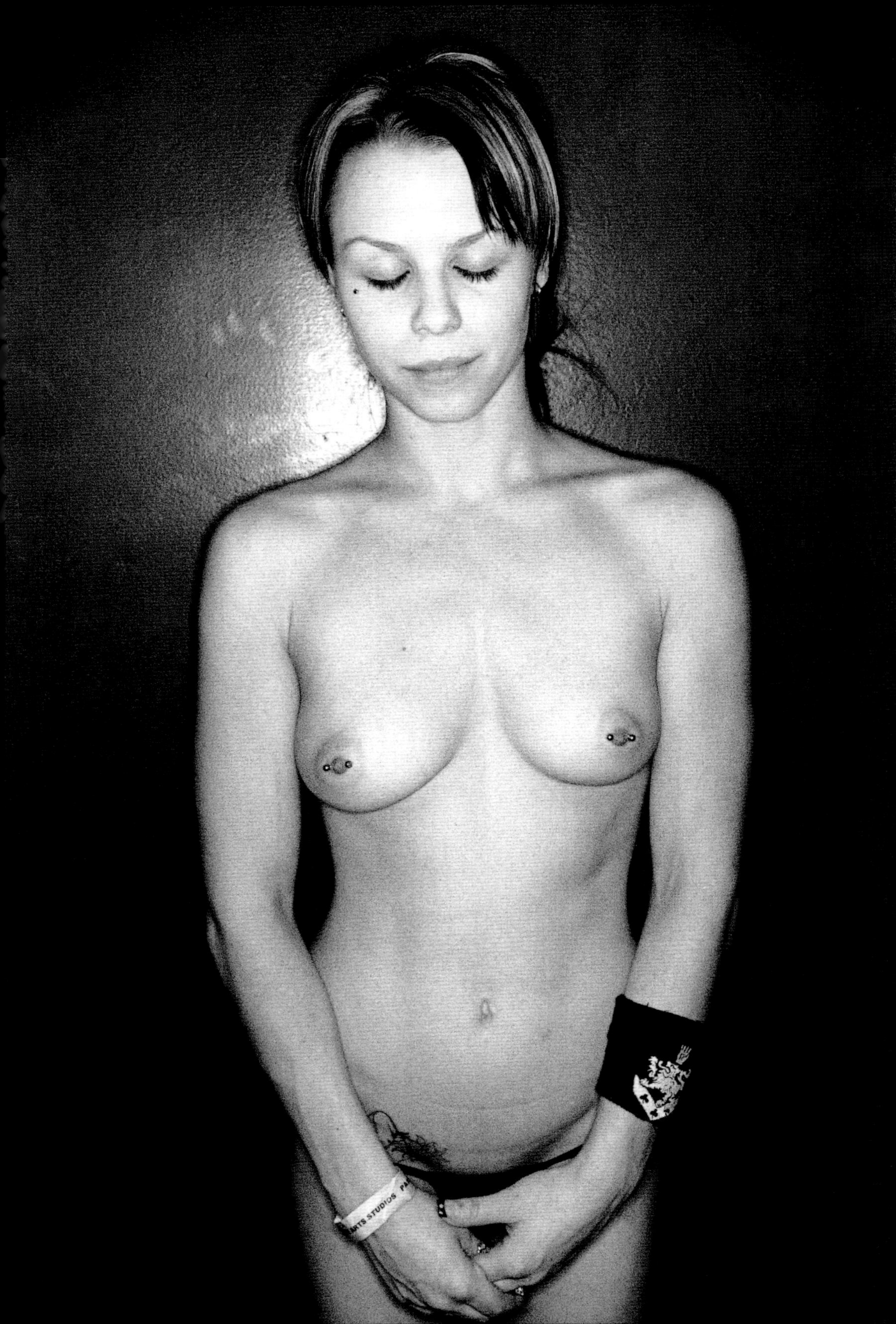

Nikki

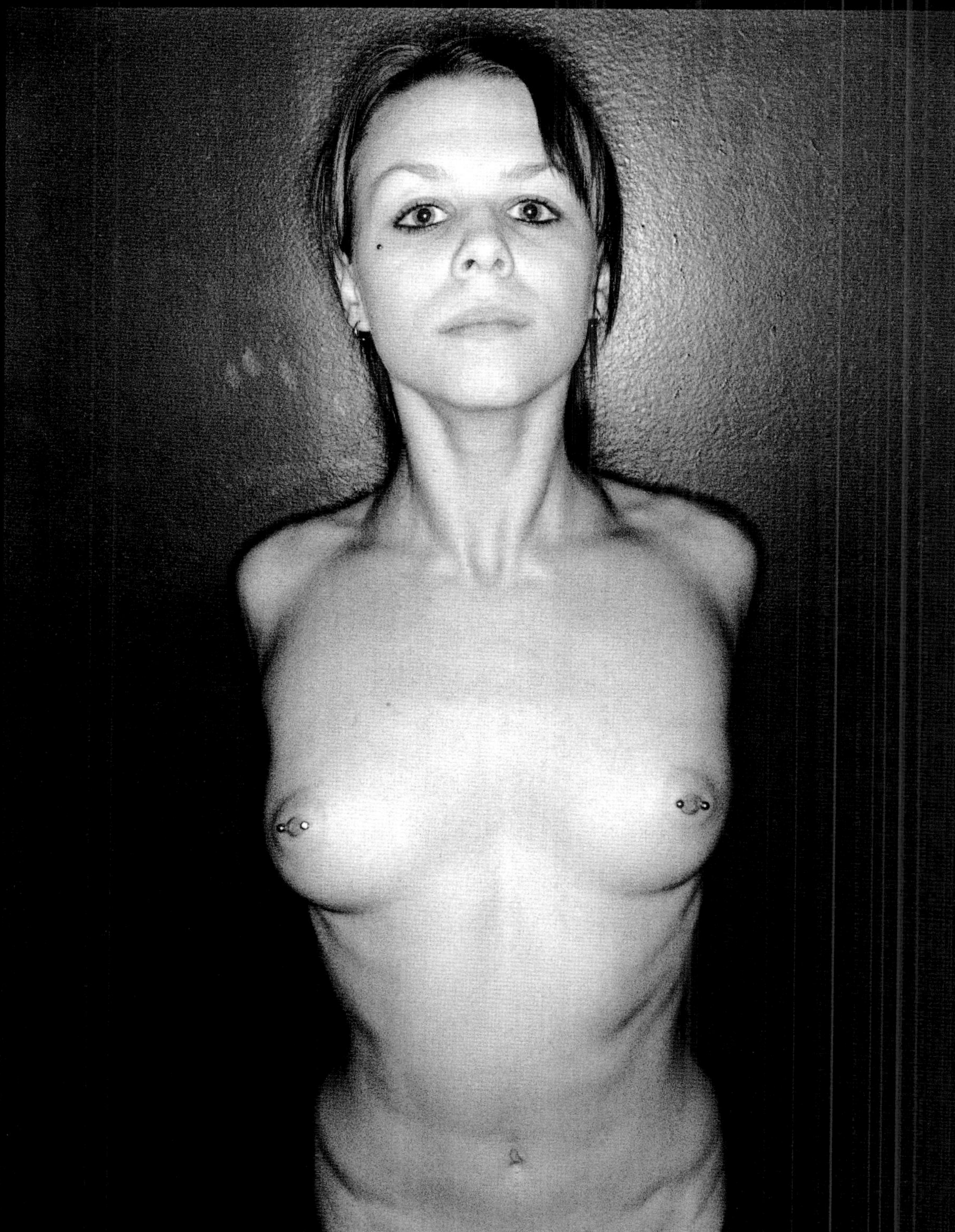

Nikki

This is the first printing of *Scar Tissue*
Photographs copyright 2010 by Assaf Pocker
Introduction copyright 2010 by Renee T. Coulombe, PhD
Gelatin silver prints by Marc Valesalla

Printed in Hong Kong
ISBN 978-1-59005-290-7

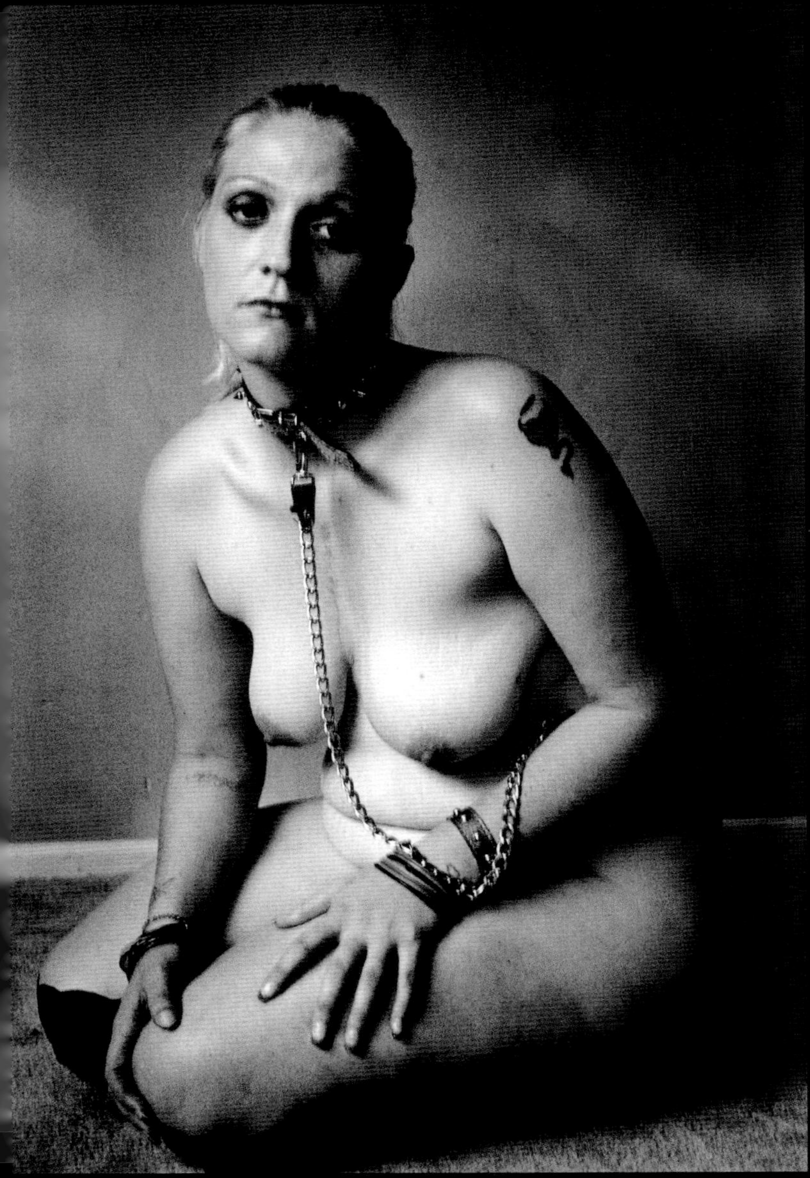

Scar Tissue is dedicated with profound gratitude to the memory of Sassy (Tawnia Dooley) * 7.13.1975 † 8.23.2007. Her heart gave in while giving birth to her daughter. Your courage and strength inspire us still.

The way of heaven is like the bending of a bow.
What is high up gets pulled down.
What is low down gets pulled up. —Tao Te Ching